Managing Madness in the Community

Critical Issues in Health and Medicine

Edited by Rima D. Apple, University of Wisconsin–Madison, and Janet Golden, Rutgers University, Camden

Growing criticism of the U.S. health care system is coming from consumers, politicians, the media, activists, and health care professionals. The Critical Issues in Health and Medicine series explores these contemporary dilemmas from political, legal, historical, sociological, and comparative perspectives, among others, with attention to crucial dimensions such as race, gender, ethnicity, sexuality, and culture.

For a list of series titles, see the last page of this book.

Managing Madness in the Community

The Challenge of Contemporary Mental Health Care

Kerry Michael Dobransky

Rutgers University Press

New Brunswick, New Jersey, and London

Library of Congress Cataloging in Publication Data

Dobransky, Kerry Michael, 1976–
    Managing madness in the community : the challenge of contemporary mental health
care / Kerry Michael Dobransky
        pages   cm. — (Critical issues in health and medicine)
    Includes bibliographical references and index
    ISBN 978–0–8135–6309–1 (hardcover : alk. paper) — ISBN 978–0–8135–6308–4
(pbk. : alk. paper) — ISBN 978–0–8135–6310–7 (e-book)
    1. Community mental health services—United States. 2. Mentally ill—Care—United
States. 3. Social integration—United States. I. Title.
    RA790.6.D63 2014
    362.2'20973—dc23
                                                                                    2013027187

A British Cataloging-in-Publication record for this book is available from the British Library.

Visit our website: http://rutgerspress.rutgers.edu

Manufactured in the United States of America

For Sarah
"By My Side"

Contents

Tables

Preface and Acknowledgments

The roots of this project can be traced to my time as a social worker. In the late 1990s and early 2000s, I worked in child welfare in a state that was participating in the Annie E. Casey Foundation's Family to Family initiative. The initiative held as its goal to build a "family-centered, neighborhood-based" child welfare system. Though the county I worked in was not part of the initiative, its principles began to diffuse there, in part under the influence of county administrators. Among the many goals of the program was a call for more active roles for parents and community members of children removed from their homes in determining what happened to those children. Because the aim of child welfare casework is often reunification—at least initially—this may not be that surprising. However, in day-to-day conversations among workers regarding the implementation of these principles, some major contradictions emerged. Children were removed from homes because of serious deficiencies in the environment there. Generally, fingers were pointed in the direction of their caregivers (usually parents). The question was asked: If this is the case, and the deficiencies are clear—usually documented in court records—why should these individuals have a say in what happens to their children until those deficiencies are acknowledged and addressed? These parents are seen as mentally or morally lacking. Child welfare workers see themselves as having the insight and training to address these problems, to care for the children, and to determine when parents should be involved again. Incorporating parents in decision-making immediately questioned this professional expertise and turned the child welfare worker-parent dynamic on its head. Ambiguity and complaints were widespread.

I later worked as a substitute house manager for a multiservice mental health care organization for people with severe mental illness. During staff meetings I was reminded of my experience in child welfare, as I encountered for the first time discussions regarding the concept of mental health recovery. In frequent discussions on the ambiguity of "recovery" in a mental health context, workers noted a fundamental contradiction in their jobs when trying to implement treatment. They were mental health professionals, experts in treating people with mental illness, yet clients likewise were to be considered "experts" in their own care, determining goals of treatment and means to achieve those goals.

As I returned to this contradiction as a research topic, I connected it to a broader push for client *empowerment* in mental health services. Since the middle of the twentieth century, concern for the rights of the subjects of human services—evident in both of my work settings—has gained rhetorical traction and also faced the hard realities of implementation. I explored those issues in two community-based nonprofit mental health organizations like the one in which I had worked. These types of organizations are increasingly common providers of care in today's system, with the role of state hospitals and other governmental providers being replaced by fluctuating public funding of private providers. I eventually detected four key forces in community care for people with severe mental illness—empowerment, professionalism, community integration, and bureaucratic forces. I came to understand them as *institutional logics* in the *field* of mental health services. At times they worked in tandem for the same means and ends, but, as I experienced on my own and confirmed in my research, they also conflicted. This project explores these conflicting situations and the ways workers deal with them.

Several colleagues have played an important role in this work from its inception. Judith Cook was gracious in her help locating and accessing appropriate sites. Michaela DeSoucey, Wendy Griswold, Eszter Hargittai, Terry McDonnell, Bernice Pescosolido, Art Stinchcombe, Berit Vannebo, and especially Carol Heimer and Corey Fields all provided invaluable early feedback, guidance, and critique. A number of others were gracious enough to lend their eyes and minds to reading drafts of chapters, even though for some the topics were not exactly their specialties: Ben Brewer, Bethany Bryson, Keo Cavalcanti, Chris Colocousis, Matt Ezzell, Allan Horwitz, Nikitah Imani, Mark Peyrot, Steve Poulson, Teresa Scheid, Celeste Watkins-Hayes, and Joe Spear. The reviewers at Rutgers were incisive and helped make a better manuscript. Peter Mickulas at Rutgers was insightful and efficient—overall a pleasure to work with. Susan Campbell's keen eye greatly benefited the manuscript. Any remaining shortcomings are solely my own responsibility. Versions of various chapters were presented at Northwestern University, University of Louisville, Loyola Marymount University, James Madison University, and the annual meetings of the American Sociological Association and the Society for the Study of Social Problems; the helpful feedback I received from all these forums was much appreciated. Earlier drafts of parts of chapter 3 were published as "The Good, the Bad, and the Severely Mentally Ill: Official and Informal Labels as Organizational Resources in Community Mental Health Services," in *Social Science and Medicine* 69 (2009):722–728; and "Labeling, Looping and Social Control:

Contextualizing Diagnosis in Mental Health Care," in *Advances in Medical Sociology* 12 (2011):111–131. They are included here with permission from Elsevier and Emerald.

As I've learned is commonly the case, the research, writing, and publishing of this project was not restricted to nine-to-five shifts in a comfy office. Thus, more thanks are in order. Generous financial support came from Northwestern University and James Madison University. The welcoming environments provided by the many cafés where much of this work was written—especially Starbucks in Rogers Park, Chicago, Illinois, and in Staunton, Virginia—were a sustaining force. The staffs of the interlibrary loan departments in the Northwestern University and James Madison University libraries were always gracious and helpful during my extensive use of their facilities. The clients and workers at both research sites were wonderfully open and welcoming to a stranger exploring their personal and professional lives. I hope the result can contribute in some way to bettering those lives. Finally, this book—along with many other aspects of my life—never would have been possible without my partner, Sarah Blythe. She is a major source of my own empowerment, mental health, and happiness.

A note on terminology: A variety of terms are used to refer to those being treated for behavioral health problems, depending on the period and the treatment setting. The terms "client," "participant," "consumer," "member," "patient," and "subject," among others, have all been used. Though a particular term may be used to highlight a point, I attempt for the most part to stick with "client," even changing words quoted from individuals without necessarily noting so in the text. I find this increases readability and helps protect confidentiality.

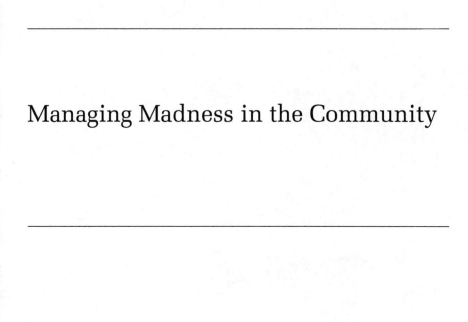

Managing Madness in the Community

Chapter 1

Introduction

Jabar Jones was pretty content with life at Suburban, a multiservice mental health care organization outside a midwestern US city. With an official diagnosis of schizoaffective disorder, he had spent the previous three decades involved with the mental health system in one form or another, including more than twenty hospitalizations. Had he been born a couple of decades earlier, Jabar could easily have spent those decades in a state hospital. Instead, coming of age and becoming ill in the era of deinstitutionalization, he fell into the all-too-familiar pattern of contemporary community care for people diagnosed with severe mental illness: residential and psychiatric instability. Having attended Suburban's day program while living at a nursing facility for a few years, Jabar made the move to Suburban's group home a few years prior to our meeting.

Compared to the alternatives he had experienced in the mental health system, living at Suburban had many advantages. All the residential programs he had been involved in had met his basic needs—food, a roof over his head, basic medical and psychiatric care—but he was given a lot more autonomy at Suburban. Two areas in particular stood out for Jabar. First, he had much more control over his money at Suburban than at the nursing facility where he had previously lived. The nursing facility was for-profit, as most are, and kept all his income except for a $30 per month allowance, which remained the same regardless of whether he supplemented his Social Security income through work or not. At Suburban, however, it was different: "Here, everything over my rent, I keep. I work . . . I get to keep all my money," he said. Jabar also liked having more control over when and how much he ate than he had in previous placements. However, not everything was positive for him or for the staff that provided him with care.

Staff members at Suburban were concerned about Jabar. He had once attended the day program and had obtained a job at a cafeteria, but he had been fired from the job and no longer regularly attended the day program. Staff claimed that since his firing, his motivation had waned. One group home staff member said, "He just lays around, eats, sleeps, and smokes cigarettes" (interview). Further, Jabar spent his money in ways that caused problems for him and for Suburban. He was months behind in paying rent. Other residents of the group home pointed out a double standard with Jabar, arguing that he was permitted to not meet his obligations while they were not allowed to do the same. On the other hand, Jabar made claims of a reverse double standard, saying staff members were holding him to a higher standard than another resident in the house who had schizophrenia.

Because Jabar was a client at a mental health services organization and had an official diagnosis of severe mental illness, one might find his problematic behaviors no big surprise. This picture of Jabar as a severely mentally ill individual was the one depicted in his clinical file, which described him as at times experiencing unspecified delusions and disordered thought processes. He was prescribed a host of medications, including antipsychotics. However, in numerous staff discussions regarding Jabar that I observed, his behavior was not described in this setting as resulting from mental illness. Rather, his disruptions were referred to as willful acts. Hence, it was a challenge to determine exactly what staff thought of Jabar's mental state. Jabar himself did not connect his current behaviors with mental illness; he discussed them as based in rational decisions. He felt the day program no longer interested him, saying, "They can't teach me nothing new" (interview). He did, however, participate in illness management and recovery, an "evidence-based practice" involving his setting goals and working with a staff member and a curriculum to achieve those goals. Among the top goals he set were losing weight and catching up on his back rent—two problems that were directly tied to the freedoms Suburban had brought him.

It became clear that staff felt pulled in a number of directions. Suburban's delivery of services (and the outcomes of those services), and their use of the resources their funders provided, was increasingly tracked and audited. This made "evidence-based" services such as illness management and recovery increasingly attractive. Impending changes in the state's Medicaid mental health financing were leading to changes for organizations like Suburban that depended on that funding. At Suburban, this meant that there was an increased pressure for staff to make sure clients were participating in activities that were Medicaid-billable. In most cases, Suburban could not bill the state for clients sitting around the group home smoking and eating—as Jabar was reported doing most of the time.

Another force at work at Suburban was a long-standing impetus to move clients out of mental health services organizations and into independence in "the community." The move Jabar had made from living in the nursing facility to Suburban's group home—a "less restrictive setting"—was a step in this direction, as was his work in the cafeteria. A further step would be his obtaining steady work and moving to an apartment, both of which Jabar expressed interest in doing. At the same time, however, he did not appear to be investing much effort in locating more work, and even he realized that with his limited income and money problems, moving out would be difficult to achieve. He said he had located and qualified for numerous apartments in the past, but he had lacked money for a deposit when they became available.

Alongside the tracking and community integration, Suburban's parent organization also had adopted the "recovery" model of mental health services. This generally meant that clients were to have a much more active role in their treatment. Thus, staff believed they were not supposed to force clients to do anything that they did not want to do when it came to treatment, and it was very rare to kick clients out of housing. It also meant that they could not arrange a behavioral contract with Jabar—a behavior modification strategy involving a written agreement between a client and an organization—though the organization had used the tool in the past.

In the midst of these other forces, staff also struggled to exercise their own "expert" judgment in how to provide services. As complaints regarding differential treatment from both Jabar and his housemates revealed, there was no "cookie cutter" approach to handling clients. Plainly put, another client in the group home was seen as much more seriously ill than he was. Thus, she was not expected to conform to rules as much as Jabar was. It was a clinical decision—the type that staff felt was increasingly difficult for them to make in the face of other forces.

What emerged was a somewhat disorganized strategy. On the one hand, an administrator directed Suburban to put Jabar under "protective payee" status with Social Security. This meant that Jabar would be deemed officially incompetent to manage his money—removing this freedom he held so dear. His Social Security checks would be sent directly to Suburban, with them having final say on how his money would be spent. Thus, they could make sure he was caught up on his rent, and the organization would receive reimbursement for services. Another policy, less formally outlined, was that some of Suburban's workers encouraged Jabar to move out of the group home of his own accord and even offered him limited financial assistance for doing so. This move toward community independence occurred despite the fact that many staff doubted his ability to manage living independently. Although they could not remove him from the organization, they *could* help him choose to remove *himself.*

Fragmentation in Mental Health Services

The above story will be all too familiar to anyone acquainted with services for people with severe, persistent mental illness (SPMI) in the United States. By all accounts, the lack of unity or coherence in American community mental health services is stark. The number of conflicting players and priorities at work in a given case or situation—the *fragmentation* of mental health services—is often overwhelming for both clients and those providing services.

Most discussions of this fragmentation describe two key divisions in the administration and financing of services for people with SPMI. The first major division is between the different levels of government involved in mental health care. Public mental health care had first been the institutional respon- sibility of local governments (through almshouses and poorhouses), then state governments (through state mental hospitals). Although the federal Veterans Administration had historically provided mental health care, it was not until the middle of the twentieth century that the federal government became more broadly involved in mental health policy (Grob 1991). The National Mental Health Act, signed in 1946, created the National Institute of Mental Health (NIMH) and the National Advisory Mental Health Council. Thus began the sustained—if at times tumultuous—large-scale partnership between federal and state governments in the development, funding, and provision of mental health care. Through providing grants-in-aid to states, and by funding demon- stration programs and clinics in states, the federal government came to take a more hands-on role in mental health care and policy. This role continued with the President John F. Kennedy's signature of the Mental Retardation Facilities and Community Mental Health Centers Act in 1963 (hereafter, CMHC program or act). Although the two thousand planned centers in the bill were not con- structed (and, indeed, the entire CMHC program was all but dismantled over time), the construction of a third of them helped to push mental health care away from its basis in state hospitals to "the community" (Grob 1991; Grob and Goldman 2007).

A true watershed in government involvement was the series of entitlement programs that finally made community care for residents of mental hospitals plausible. The creation of Social Security Disability Insurance (SSDI) in 1956, Medicaid and Medicare in 1965, and Supplemental Security Income for the Aged, the Disabled, and the Blind (SSI) in 1972 together provided the possibility that the care and general material support that patients received in the mental hospital might be replicated in the community. SSDI serves people fifty years old or older who cannot work because of a physical or mental condition, whereas SSI provides financial support for those of any age who cannot work by virtue of age or disability. Finally, Medicaid and Medicare fund health care for the indigent and aged, respectively. Medicaid, in particular, has become a major source of funding of mental health services for people with SPMI (Day 2006; Mechanic 2007). NIMH and (since 1992) the Substance Abuse and Mental Health Services Administration (SAMHSA) continue to play a major part in the development of mental health services, funding research and demonstration programs at the national, state, and local levels.

Federal, state, and local governments all had a hand in mental health care, but what was missing was an all-encompassing oversight body. No one level of government clearly was in the driver's seat when it came to mental health services. Though the federal government played a powerful role in the overall trend toward deinstitutionalization and community care (through the CMHC act and later through the Community Support Program), states had (and still have) a great deal of autonomy in how they constructed and funded mental health services within their borders.

Overlying the fragmentation by level of government is the other type of fragmentation: among the many target categories of social, medical, and mental health policy into which members of this population fall (Dill 2001). The disability and chronicity that characterizes SPMI renders those suffering from it in need of a broad range of supports to manage life in the community successfully. Vocational services, income support, housing assistance, social rehabilitation, and health care, as well as mental health services such as medication management and counseling, are all frequently needed services (Cook and Wright 1995; Cuddeback and Morrissey 2010). However, policy has generally been constructed to support each of these categories of problems individually, not as an overarching whole. Each category has distinct eligibility criteria, and each may be administered or financed from a different level of government—or from more than one level at the same time. The lack of institutionalized communication channels and coordination could lead, at one extreme, to many clients "falling through the cracks," and at the other, to duplication of services. The tasks of determining which "slots" a given person falls into, and of managing the varying demands raised by membership in each, can be challenging for even the savviest client or worker.

This problem has led to a number of efforts at "integrating services" in mental health care (and health care and social services more broadly) (Cuddeback and Morrissey 2010; Kagan, Neville, and National Center for Service Integration 1993; Kahn and Kamerman 1992). For instance, the Robert Wood Johnson–sponsored Program on Chronic Mental Illness (PCMI) and the SAMHSA-funded Access to Community Care and Effective Services and Supports (ACCESS) demonstration programs both focused on integrating services for people with SPMI. The goals of the initiatives were to integrate services not only to improve coordination and efficiency, but also to improve mental health outcomes for those involved. Whereas the PCMI focused on integration of services for people with SPMI generally, the ACCESS program focused specifically on homeless individuals with SPMI. Though both programs were successful at achieving a better integrated system and improving access to services for clients, there were not significant improvements in mental health outcomes for those clients in the integrated settings (Lehman et al. 1994; Rosenheck et al. 1998; Rosenheck et al. 2002; Rothbard et al. 2004). However, another set of integrated services, service models that integrate treatment for clients with dual diagnoses of substance abuse and SPMI (who thus fall into two distinct categories of need), has been effectively implemented and is currently seen as one of a handful of established "evidence-based practices" in mental health services (Drake et al. 2001a; Drake et al. 2001b). Unfortunately, such successful outcomes are narrow in scope, and rare. These disappointing overall results led the head commissioner of the President's New Freedom Commission on Mental Health to state unequivocally that "systems integration is not the answer" to curing what ails the mental health system (quoted in Grob and Goldman 2007:175).

Examining Jabar's situation at Suburban provides insight into why focusing on service fragmentation may not tell the whole story. There is no doubt that service fragmentation existed for clients at Suburban. For instance, the group home Jabar lived in was funded through a program of the federal Department of Housing and Urban Development (HUD); most mental health services provided at Suburban's day program were funded through state/federal Medicaid funds. The two programs had some distinct eligibility requirements. Medicaid, which is tied to federal SSI eligibility, requires documentation of mental disability, whereas some HUD programs require documentation of homelessness and financial need. However, Jabar (and Suburban) depended on his SSI income to make up the balance of his HUD-subsidized rent. Vocational services Jabar received from Suburban in the past were paid for through the state's Division of Rehabilitation Services and were thus subject to that program's guidelines and eligibility criteria. Suburban therefore needed to work with (or at times against) Jabar to patch together resources from a dizzying array of different categorical and governmental sources to fund services for him.

However, though we have evidence of service fragmentation, fragmentation alone does not sufficiently explain core features of Suburban's situation. Some of the major forces pulling staff and Jabar in different directions were bound neither to one level of government nor to one categorical service sector—they transcended them. For example, bureaucratic accountability, the driving force behind much of the push for tracking and billable services described above, can be found in demands from consumers, private foundations, and governmental bodies in a range of sectors of society (Strathern 2000)—from education (Hallett 2010) and law (Espeland and Vannebo 2007) to health care (Mendel and Scott 2010; Scott et al. 2000) and mental health care (Manderscheid, Henderson, and Brown 2001). Similarly, calls for empowerment evident in the recovery movement Suburban embraced are rooted in the civil rights movement of the 1960s but have since spread to mental health "consumers" (McLean 2000) and to consumers more generally (Cohen 2003). Two other major forces compelling workers at Suburban can be found in the move toward client independence in the community and the workers' push for respecting their own expert judgment, both also evident in Jabar's situation described above.

I show that each of these forces is an *institutional logic*, "a set of material practices and symbolic constructions [that] constitutes the organizing principles" of the health care and social services fields (Friedland and Alford 1991: 248). Basically, the logic dictates how the setting works—or should work. Some logics are associated with each of the major institutional orders of society—capitalism, democracy, the state, family, religion—and others are more specific, covering certain sectors of society such as academic publishing (Thornton and Ocasio 1999), manufacturing (Greenwood et al. 2010), or health care (Scott et al. 2000).

There are multiple logics at play in any institutional setting, and they interact and compete with one another. Although one logic may be dominant in a given period, over time another may displace it without eliminating it completely (Thornton and Ocasio 2008). For instance, Peter Mendel, W. Richard Scott, and colleagues examine the shift in the health care field since the 1940s, tracing the dominant logics across four eras (Mendel and Scott 2010; Scott et al. 2000).

They argue that the logics of "professional authority" and "quality of care" held sway during the mid-twentieth century. Beginning in the 1960s, this was supplanted by an era in which a logic of "equity of access" dominated. Importantly, during this era the entry of government involvement through Medicare, Medicaid, and other regulations, alongside the already existing private system, led to fragmentation. Beginning in the 1980s another era began, in which existing logics were overlain by a "managerial-market" logic, which became dominant. Here, efficiency, reduced costs, and increased profits were major focuses. Finally, since 2000, the authors argue, we have entered an era in which the dominant logic is "value-based services," the belief that "expenditures on health services should be consonant with benefits"—what I refer to (combining elements of the dominant logics of these last two eras) as the logic of bureaucratic accountability (Mendel and Scott 2010: 258). Once again, however, previous logics have not been eliminated; they exist alongside and compete with this logic, leading to "institutional complexity" (Greenwood et al. 2010).

In this book, I describe four major institutional logics in the mental health services field: the clinical-professional logic, the community logic, the empowerment logic, and the logic of bureaucratic accountability. Within any contemporary mental health services setting, all four logics will be present to a degree, though they vary in dominance at any given time. Further, I show how they conflict, pulling workers and clients in many directions, fragmenting priorities and protocols in the service setting. I refer to this situation as *institutional fragmentation*. There are two senses in which I use the concept fragmentation. The first is *fragmentation in meaning*. Part of the function of institutional logics is to give organizational members a system of schemas to make sense of their experiences. How organizational reality is divided and classified changes depending on the logic applied (Thornton and Ocasio 2008). With competing logics, workers are beset with a range of possible meanings and classifications and must choose which to apply if there are conflicts. For instance, in a given situation at Suburban or Urban (the other field site, which is discussed below), a client might be 1) a mentally ill individual in need of clinical intervention (clinical-professional); 2) a person working toward living in a less restrictive environment (community); 3) an expert in his/her own care (empowerment); or 4) a source of billable hours (bureaucratic accountability). If the client did not want to take medication, for example, the first and third classifications would likely conflict.

Another closely related sense in which I discuss workers experiencing institutional fragmentation is *fragmentation in decision-making*. In both formal and informal settings, workers have to decide where to direct their attention (Ocasio 1997) and to make decisions about clients and about organizational life and their own place within it. Further, these logics may not have one or more clearly defined representatives in the organizations; the institutional logics that are the focus of my analysis cut across many stakeholders and, in many cases, did not have clear representatives. Calling on W. Richard Scott's (2008) institutional "pillars" of social life—regulative, normative, and cultural-cognitive—I focus on the *type of institutionalization* of each of the logics in understanding their relative influence on organizational decision-making. For an actor in an organizational field—for example, a worker in a mental health care organization—each of these different types of institutionalization is experienced as a distinct form of constraint on his or her thought or action, narrowing what is considered acceptable or possible in a given setting or situation.

The first type of institutionalization is *regulative*, in which the key values and practices of an institution are translated in the formal rules and regulations of the field. Thus, actors have concrete limits placed upon their action, forcing them to either embrace fully and comply with the regulations or, at the very least, give "ceremonial" adherence to them while actually pursuing other goals (often referred to as "loose coupling") (Meyer and Rowan 1977). The second type is *normative*, in which components of a logic become infused with value and are experienced as a duty to comply with. Publicly violating a normatively institutionalized element "resembles a taboo rather than the infraction of rules" (Schneiberg and Clemens 2006:213). Finally, with *cultural-cognitive* institutionalization, elements are taken for granted, "sedimented" into an actor's fundamental understanding of reality; alternatives are nearly incomprehensible (or at least highly implausible). Because they are so unquestioned, elements of organizational life embedded this way are rarely explicitly articulated and are best observed in noting "silences," those aspects of life that are shared and acted upon but are not discussed or noted by actors (Schneiberg and Clemens 2006). I show that the degree to which a given logic is institutionalized in a particular manner affects how it plays out in practice and how it interacts with other logics, which might be embedded differently.

Logics penetrate and embed in organizations in different ways and to different degrees. Calling on symbolic interactionist approaches to organizations, I focus on the locally negotiated character of patterns of decision-making (Barley 2008; Hallett and Ventresca 2006; Strauss et al. 1963). Members of an organization, facing the constraints the various logics pose, negotiate the means to meet, balance, or work around various demands and make organizational life

function. When combined with service fragmentation, this institutional fragmentation can render mental health care a morass, one in which workers and
clients must manage conflicting demands not only from different stakeholders,
but also at times even from *the same* stakeholder.

State government, for example—a major stakeholder in public mental
health services—imposed both the empowerment logic and the logic of bureaucratic accountability on Suburban. Regarding the former, the state government
took a cue from the report of the federal President's New Freedom Commission
on Mental Health, which held as one of its central goals that mental health services be "consumer and family driven" (President's New Freedom Commission
on Mental Health 2003). Suburban's state performed a wide-ranging evaluation
of public mental health services. The resulting report recommended, in part,
making services within the state "consumer and family driven." Key to this was
making the system more "recovery-oriented" and giving consumers "choice in
treatment." Another state document defining the principles of recovery stated
that a core measure of success in implementing recovery was clients acting
on their right to make independent choices regarding their own community
engagement, personal, social, monetary, or vocational goals. In line with this
perspective, Suburban's parent organization, Wellness, had an administrative-
level client recovery staff member, herself a mental health consumer, who
worked to train staff and implement recovery-oriented services. From this perspective, Jabar should have been able to decline participation in the day program and household activities, as that was his choice.

However, at the same time, the state also made clear that there were only
certain things for which it would reimburse mental health care organizations
providing particular services. As many states were doing even before the widespread budget crises of the Great Recession, this state government (already in
dire financial straits) worked to reduce health care and social service expenditures. A strategy applied in so doing was to restrict and more closely monitor
its reimbursements to mental health providers. As part of this effort, the state
rolled out a new set of Medicaid service definitions and a new fee-for-service
payment system during my study. At one staff meeting, Suburban's director
said that, in conversations with the state's mental health department, he and
other directors had been told that their clients should not be sitting idle in the
lounge area of the program for extended periods, nor should they be absent
from the program regularly. Because one of the primary mental health services
Suburban provided was psychosocial rehabilitation—which the mental health
department defined as a "high-intensity" activity—clients should be present

and actively engaged if they were enrolled in the day program. Thus, staff members were encouraged to "motivate" clients to be more involved. If clients did not comply, the organization could "boot" them from the program, telling them, "you're in the wrong program" (field notes). Within this context, Jabar's extremely sporadic attendance and lack of engagement at the day program was not acceptable—nor was his idleness around the group home. Thus, from the same stakeholder—the state—staff had to contend with two different institutional imperatives in dealing with problematic clients such as Jabar. As will be shown, because the logic of bureaucratic accountability was more thoroughly institutionalized in regulation than the empowerment logic, workers were more likely to act on that logic when this type of institutional fragmentation occurred.

This book focuses on these types of conflicting institutional demands as experienced in organizations that provide mental health care for people with SPMI. It examines the character of the logics and looks into how they are experienced and dealt with in the actual service setting. Workers and clients must navigate and adapt to the constraints and imperatives the different logics bring, developing their own strategies to do so. In the next section, I discuss in more detail the two organizations that were the focus of this study.

Methods and Setting

The data for this study come from a fifteen-month organizational ethnography, conducted in 2006 and 2007. The setting is two multiservice mental health care organizations for individuals with SPMI in a metropolitan area in the midwestern region of the United States. For much of the time in the field, I attended meetings, treatment groups, and counseling sessions. During periods of idle time, I talked informally and played games with workers and clients. Semi-structured interviews with forty-two clients and forty-nine workers supplement the ethnographic data. In the interviews, I pushed both clients and workers to reflect critically on statements and behaviors I witnessed during the course of observation. Interviews lasted from twenty minutes to two hours, averaging approximately one hour. I also collected documents, both those used by and those produced by the organizations. These included policy and procedure materials produced by government and the organizations themselves, materials posted on walls, and materials used in treatment groups. Finally, both clients and the organizations granted me access to the complete clinical files of thirty-nine clients (all but three of the forty-two I interviewed). These files included clinical treatment plans and day-to-day clinical notes produced by the organizations, as well as collateral reports produced by and for other service providers. Data were coded and analyzed using a grounded theory approach, involving an iterative interplay between data collection and analysis (Strauss 1987). Field notes were analyzed using the qualitative data analysis program ATLAS.ti. The institutional review boards of Northwestern University and those of both organizations studied provided ethical approval of the research design. In order to protect respondents' and organizations' identities, all names used are pseudonyms, and identifying information has been altered or omitted. The excerpts or quotations reported in the text are, unless otherwise noted, selected because they are representative of patterns I found in the data.

The first site, which I refer to as "Urban," comprised the mental health and substance abuse services programs of a larger organization. Located in a gentrifying neighborhood in a Midwestern city, Urban's main building sat on a busy corner in an area with a number of health and human services providers. This led to an interesting combination of people surrounding the building. Although urban "hipsters" and young professionals frequently passed, they were usually on their way to some other destination. People who were more likely to use the organization's services—the homeless, the unemployed, the symptomatic, or other needy populations—were likely to spend longer periods of time standing outside the organization's building. Throughout its various programs, Urban served about three hundred clients; most were African American and most were men. There were approximately fifty staff members, a little over half of whom were White, split evenly along gender lines. The most common psychiatric diagnoses of clients here were psychotic disorders such as schizophrenia, or severe mood disorders such as bipolar disorder or major depression.

Urban's building was old, and its age showed. During my time there, it served a couple of functions: several divisions of Urban's parent organization (including mental health and addiction services and a primary health clinic) operated there, and there were also residential apartments rented to the general public on some floors. Entrances to the two areas were segregated so that residents could largely avoid clients and workers inside the building. Urban's clients were frequently reminded of this division by the building's security guard. Clients and workers generally took an elevator to Urban's areas. Should clients become tired of waiting for the elevator and opt to take the stairs instead, they would be disappointed to find that the door to the day program's floor was locked from the inside (locking from both sides presumably violated the fire code)—this was apparently done in an attempt to discourage illicit activity from taking place in the stairwell.

The case management and outreach staff were on different floors from the day program and its staff.[1] Clients were usually encouraged to participate in both programs, though not all did. The day program, behind a door that was kept closed during operating hours and locked at all other times, was relatively small: there was a lounging area with chairs and tables, a boom box, and a few computers. There was also an area for cooking food—with a stove, sink, refrigerator, and cabinets with food—and a clothes washer and dryer. Down the hallway at the far end of the room were bathrooms and staff offices. Walls throughout the building were adorned with client artwork completed during art groups. In all of Urban's programs, the physical environment was quite spartan. Few of the items in the buildings appeared newly purchased, though they were generally functional. Image seemed less important than mission—resources were directed to providing services, not to looking good while doing so.

On an average day, around forty clients attended the day program (with the highest numbers—during parties—reaching a little over one hundred). The day generally began with staff reporting to work an hour before the program opened to clients. Clients lined up outside the door to the program, waiting for it to open. When the door opened, they entered and snatched up the fruit and coffee laid out for them. They then used the telephone, washer, and other facilities. Some would attend groups—often with some staff prodding—while others simply rested on the couches or chairs, resting places that were often hard for clients to find in public (most shelters, where many clients stayed, forced their residents to leave at 5:30 A.M. Groups covered a variety of psychosocial and substance abuse topics, with names such as Substance Abuse Management and Relationships. Attendance at the program peaked around lunchtime—lunch was free and was the only meal of the day for some clients. There were generally no tightly enforced rules for group attendance, so clients made those choices for themselves. After lunch, many—if not most—clients left, even though groups continued and the program was open for at least another hour. After the last client left and the day program closed, staff completed paperwork and, at some point, gathered to "debrief" regarding any notable issues that arose during the day.

The case management program worked a bit differently. Because staff members in this program were supposed to visit clients in clients' "natural setting," much work happened outside Urban's building. Although clients and case management staff might meet briefly in the day program area, staff often visited clients in their place of residence (if they had one) or other "community" location. Visits could cover virtually any issue, from cleanliness of the clients' homes to medication issues to relationships with family and friends to substance abuse. Often, however, the clients' major concern was receiving their Social Security benefits checks—frequently the clients' sole source of income—which Urban was in many instances designated by the government to distribute to clients. If they did not yet have Social Security benefits, the organizations would work with clients to try to obtain them.

The second site, which I refer to as "Suburban," was located outside the same city. Constituting one self-standing program in a larger organization, Suburban provided vocational services, including a sheltered workshop (where clients did light assembly work in Suburban's building on a flexible schedule for sub-minimum wages) and a full range of community mental health services. All clients served by Suburban had to come to the building for services, which included psychosocial rehabilitation, job services, case management, and psychiatric services. Suburban also ran one group home. Most of the one hundred clients were White, as were most staff members. Half of the clients were men; women made up the majority of the approximately fifteen-person staff.

Situated in a neighborhood interspersed with small industrial and residential properties, the organization's building fell into the former category. Foot traffic outside the building was minimal—mainly people walking to or from their cars to nearby businesses. Suburban's building comprised two major areas: one containing offices, meeting rooms, and a lunchroom and a kitchen; the other a combined workshop and warehouse area. Unlike Urban's kitchen, which included appliances that might have been found in a household, Suburban's kitchen was equipped with restaurant-size, professional-grade appliances. The décor of the building as a whole did not match the degree of luxury found in the kitchen: the furnishings, although not as "used" as the furnishings at Urban, were by no means opulent.

Here both the case management and treatment groups were handled by the same staff members. Each staff member had an individual caseload in addition to a certain number of groups, which ran on a "quarter" system (compared with Urban, where groups ran continuously). Groups covered a range of topics such as medications, sexuality, thinking skills, and employment skills. At the end of each quarter, clients received an evaluation of their performance in the group and the entire schedule of groups would change. Clients who came to Suburban generally had to be transported there by vehicle, either through public or private means. Most clients lived either with family or in nursing facilities, and thus had a higher level of resources available to them than clients at Urban, where the organization was often clients' sole or main source of support.

In addition to the day program's mental health services, there was a major vocational component to the program as well. This included a couple of full-time vocational staff members, with other workers contributing. Vocational staff assisted clients in finding jobs outside the organization and oversaw clients working in the sheltered workshop. The workshop used to run as a fully functioning business, with a range of customers. When the workshop merged with the day program, however, and came under the purview of Suburban's parent organization, less emphasis was placed on the workshop as a business (and as a part of the program overall). Thus, less effort was made to find customers and to make sure there was sufficient staffing to meet customer demands. Clients worked when they felt like it instead of adhering to a strict schedule. Nevertheless, there was a tight contingent of very dedicated clients who spent large chunks of time in the workshop nearly every day the program was open. At the end of my research, plans were under way to eliminate the workshop altogether.

The day program at Suburban ran longer than that at Urban; it started at 8:30 A.M. and ended at 3:30 P.M. Between fifteen and twenty clients came to the organization on an average day. Clients generally arrived in groups, based on common residence or transportation source. Coffee was available upon their arrival, but food usually was not. A few times a week, the day began with a "community meeting" where staff and clients made announcements, delivered congratulations, and performed similar activities. Other days, there were "coordination" meetings, where smaller groups of clients checked in with individual staff regarding their schedule that day. After these meetings, some clients went straight to the workshop area and began working. Other clients participated in groups. Lunch here cost $1.50 unless clients worked, either making lunch or cleaning up afterward. Unlike at Urban, most clients stayed after lunch—if for no other reason than because their ride was not scheduled to arrive until the program closed and they were too far from home to walk. Vocational staff worked more flexible schedules, meeting with some clients in the program and visiting others on the job "in the community."

Within the "specialty mental health care sector," where those with more serious mental illness receive their care, multiservice mental health care organizations such as Urban and Suburban are the most common providers of nonresidential care (Milazzo-Sayre et al. 2001) (though both organizations I studied did offer additional residential services for some clients). Moreover, Medicaid-funded services such as those provided by these organizations are used by more than half of the mental health consumers served nationally by

US states (Lutterman et al. 2009) and are particularly used by the most severely mentally ill (Mechanic 2007). These organizations are thus representative of a large segment of the mental health system that serves people with SPMI in the United States today.

I selected these particular organizations because, although they are subject to many of the same institutional constraints, their differing locations result in demographics, and even some of the presenting problems of their clientele, that vary starkly (though clients at both have severe mental illness). The variation introduced by the organizations' different settings and clientele thus allows a more powerful illustration of how logics affect mental health practice.

Layout of the Book

Chapter 2 takes a deeper look into the four dominant logics in mental health services for people with SPMI: the clinical-professional logic, the empowerment logic, the community logic, and the logic of bureaucratic accountability. I outline the key components of each and show how each is institutionalized in the mental health system and the daily mental health practice of each organization. I connect the broad institutional issues to ground-level casework practice and worker-client interaction.

Chapter 3 examines the role that workers' official and informal labeling of clients plays in organizational life. I show how official labels and informal labels serve different purposes and different logics. Official labels of client mental illness tie in to the demands of the logic of bureaucratic accountability. These official labels bring resources to clients and to the organizations. Because of this, both workers and clients are apt to apply them even when there are questions regarding their validity. Informal labels of clients—regarding both client mental illness and how disruptive clients are—help workers use the clinical-professional logic in a more valid way to manage everyday organizational life. One way they do so is through determining how workers respond to clients when clients violate organizational rules and routines. The chapter also shows how official and informal labels can conflict with each other.

Chapter 4 investigates client empowerment more closely, noting that though the logic was highly valued, it was translated into few clear guidelines for frontline workers. This gave them some discretion, but staff faced a couple of different constraints in implementing empowerment. The first was variation within the client group, with some having more resources through their wealth or personal connections or through involvement in the underground economy. This made it possible for some clients to have more self-determination than others and to channel more of the providers' resources to themselves. Second were imperatives from the logic of bureaucratic accountability that conflicted with those from the empowerment logic, leading to institutional fragmentation. The chapter describes the strategies of "practical empowerment" that staff used to deal with these constraints and still implement the empowerment logic.

Chapter 5 explores the realities of community life for clients at both sites. It shows how the assumptions underlying the community logic, which was endorsed by many workers and policymakers, were not equally applicable to all clients. Clients' lived experience of community, including the community found in the mental health care organizations, was given insufficient attention. The ideal of integration into the external community could be derailed by both the draw of dysfunctional segments of that community with which clients were familiar and by clients' negative experiences in their attempts to integrate. These issues could drive clients to prefer integration into the organization's internal community. This preference set up institutional fragmentation between the community logic and the empowerment logic when clients chose dependence on the organization.

Chapter 6 takes a closer look at institutional fragmentation in staffing and finds that hiring was fragmented between the empowerment logic and clinical logic. Both were valued, but each was captured in separate and unequal positions within the organizations. Clinically trained staff held higher-status positions; those without clinical training, who were more frequently hired because they shared client characteristics such as mental illness, substance abuse, or race or age, held lower positions. This led to distinct ways of interacting with and judging clients. Clinically trained workers tended to erect strict boundaries with clients and were more likely to medicalize client behavior. Workers without clinical training presented an authentic persona to clients, basing interaction on shared experiences, and were more likely to moralize client behavior.

In addition to synthesizing the main arguments, the conclusion highlights the implications for research on organizations and mental health services. In order to understand organizational practice—including human services delivery—attention must be paid to dominant logics and how those logics are institutionalized. Within human services policy and practice, such a focus allows us to detect true policy priorities and to distinguish between mere rhetoric and real regulatory heft.

Chapter 2

Logic and Constraint

Four institutional logics were dominant organizing features of day-to-day life in the mental health system in which Urban and Suburban operated, shaping how workers interpreted situations and what they did in them. However, the meanings and behavioral imperatives of the logics did not always line up. Each had its own history, stakeholders, and set of priorities in relation to client care. This chapter examines each of the logics and how they are experienced by frontline workers.

The logics varied in how and to what degree they were embedded in organizational life. Though all were to some degree institutionalized in regulation, they differed markedly in degree. Regulative institutionalization was evident when an element of the logic was included in the governing rules and policies of the field or organization. Frequently this was in the form of state policy documents governing the organizations, especially regulations covering reimbursement for Medicaid-funded services. There was also considerable variation in the amount of normative institutionalization. This form was perceptible when components of a logic took on a moral imperative—where not complying with the logic was seen as taboo and a moral failing—with support taking on an almost religious character. Examples of this were found in government or organizational statements identifying goals, values, or "visions." Most difficult to uncover was cultural-cognitive institutionalization, where the logic was taken for granted and unquestioned. Here the focus turned to what was assumed, what was not said. These logics were institutionalized at different levels of the mental health system, but in each case penetrated the organization to some

Table 2.1. Major Logics in Community Mental Health Care

	Main components	Types of institutionalization
Clinical-professional logic	Discretion, jurisdiction, expertise	Regulative, normative
Empowerment logic	Client self-determination, removal of barriers/provision of resources, peer support	(Weakly) regulative, normative
Community logic	Integration with "the natural," client independence	Regulative, cultural-cognitive
Logic of bureaucratic accountability	Documentation, standardization, productivity	Regulative, normative

degree, affecting frontline mental health practice. Put another way, focusing on the types of institutionalization outlines *how* the mental health field led workers to act or think in ways that conformed to the given logic. Before examining the conflicts between the logics, however, we need a fuller understanding of each. Table 2.1 highlights the main points of the argument that follows.

The Clinical-Professional Logic

The mental health services sector is populated by a wide range of professionals and para-professionals (Dill 2001; Hasenfeld 1986). Urban and Suburban employed people from a range of educational backgrounds, from those whose formal education ended with a GED or high school degree to those with a bachelor's degree or graduate degrees. College majors ranged from the expected concentrations in psychology, social work, counseling, nursing, and sociology to the fields of music, art, and communications. In all but a few cases, any graduate degrees workers possessed or were pursuing were in the fields of counseling, psychology, nursing, or social work. In addition to these educational credentials, a number of workers had or were pursuing licensure or certification, including LCPC (Licensed Clinical Professional Counselor), LSW (Licensed Social Worker), RN (Registered Nurse), APN (Advanced Practice Nurse), and CACD (Certified Alcohol and Drug Counselor).

Given this diversity, one might think that any unifying logic would be impossible. Nonetheless, there were several forces that together institutionalized a consistent orientation to dealing with clients that I refer to as the *clinical-professional logic*. This logic involved transforming the flow of client experiences and issues into clinical problems to be "diagnosed," "inferred," and "treated" by staff (Abbott 1988). It also dictated an unequal relationship between the client and the staff member (or human services "professional"), with staff assumed to have knowledge the client lacked (often formal, specialized, abstract knowledge) that was relevant to the client's problems (Abbott 1988; Freidson 2001). Thus, staff members were seen as rightly put in charge of handling clients' problems and of determining how and when the client should be incorporated into the decision-making process.

Main Components

A key component of being a professional at Urban and Suburban was the *discretion* allowed to workers to apply their professional skill and knowledge to a given client or situation and to react however they best saw fit. In human services, even with the lack of dominance by a single, powerful profession, the structure of the bureaucracy can result in workers having more discretion in their work with clients (Lipsky 1980; Watkins-Hayes 2009). In fact, that discretion is unavoidable, as rules and procedures can never cover every contingency (Maynard-Moody and Musheno 2003). Discretion was valued by staff, and workers believed it should be maximized, because they believed they knew how best to do their jobs. Efforts to impose standards or policies that removed that discretion were often bristled at. Workers in both organizations repeatedly reminded clients and each other that it was important to take each case and client individually, avoiding blanket policies whenever possible. At a community meeting in the day program at Urban, a staff member named Steve pointed out that staff might react differently to one client than they would to another for the same infractions. Steve said, "It's our responsibility to make this a safe place to be." He asserted that in doing so, they have to make some tough decisions. Sometimes they had to hospitalize people. Sometimes they had to ask people to leave the program. Sometimes they had to restrict privileges. He said each case is decided on an individual basis. So, at times, two people might have done the same thing, but have different "consequences" for it. He asked why that might be. One client replied that the one person might be "retractable" [redirectible] wheras the other was not. Steve agreed. He also said that one might have "been warned" several times or had the same behavior over and over again, which might result in harsher "consequences." "If you don't follow staff direction, you could receive consequences" (field notes). Steve worked with clients in this instance to unpack the staff's decision-making process, but what is most relevant here is that staff had the professional discretion to make those judgments. Similarly, at Suburban, clients and some staff noted differences in treatment between a severely symptomatic client living in the group home and other clients. Each time, a manager would remind them that "each client is unique" and that they could not compare across clients—clinical discretion needed to be respected (field notes).

Another key component of the logic that workers experienced was *jurisdiction.* For professionals, an important aspect of work is the perception that some problems are solely theirs to deal with (Abbott 1988). At Urban and Suburban, I found that, in practice, there were two claims to professional jurisdiction. First, there was a professional hierarchy in which only those with certain credentials or experience could qualify for certain government-defined positions and, in turn, perform certain tasks. Simply put, with few exceptions, those in charge, who reviewed and "signed off" (both literally and figuratively) on what was done by the lower-ranked, had more credentials or clinical experience than those below them. These workers generally had an advanced degree, certification, licensure, more than a decade providing mental health services, or any combination thereof.

The second way claims to jurisdiction were discharged in daily practice was in what one might call inter- and intra-professional "courtesy." Workers both within and across organizations were to respect the judgment of other professionals in dealing with clients. These types of claims were most commonly observed when perceived as being violated. For instance, at Suburban, many staff members who worked with clients treated by psychiatrists outside the organization claimed that those doctors did not consult or communicate well enough with the organization. One worker explained that although she sent monthly progress reports religiously to the psychiatrists, few sent any back to her. Among those that were sent, few were legible (field notes). Similarly, at a staff meeting, a few workers discussed a psychiatrist with whom they disagreed about a client. The psychiatrist's impression was that the client's symptoms and mental state were much better than staff at Suburban thought they were: "Glenda says they've had a staffing with a psychiatrist 'that just doesn't get it.' She says that there is no improvement [in the client's mental status], asking, 'Has anyone seen improvement?' [No one has] . . . Brandy says the psychiatrist sees [the client] for two minutes and says she's highly intelligent. Barry says that 'sounds good.' Brandy says, 'But then he generalizes that'" (field notes). The implication here is that the psychiatrist did not have sufficient contact and experience with the client to make the call he was making, and was not giving enough weight to the staff at Suburban's (more extensive) contact with the client in reaching his judgment. Such inter-professional problems are quite consequential with the fragmentation in services common for people with SPMI, who can receive care from a wide range of professionals and organizations. Communication and consultation can affect which services and opportunities clients are given access to—or pushed into. There was also some tension inside Suburban's walls between workers. Staff raised concerns that some workers were doing work with clients formally assigned to others. At Urban, claims of this sort were usually restricted to grumbling between different programs. I most frequently observed this type of sniping between the day program workers and the case management staff regarding not taking into consideration each others' needs or opinions.

A final key component of the clinical-professional logic as experienced at Suburban and Urban was *expertise.* There was an assumption that workers at Suburban and Urban had knowledge and experience that clients lacked and were therefore in a position to tell clients what clients should do in most circumstances. Generally, this expertise was seen as grounded in abstract psychotherapeutic knowledge in which staff members had some sort formal training. Some staff interventions with clients were geared to pointing out to them a clinical reality that they themselves were assumed to be unable to perceive. Phillip, a client at Suburban, for example, had been told by psychiatrists for years that much of what he experienced and believed (including that he was severely abused as a child) was nothing more than symptoms of his illness: "I take medication for the voices. The medication doesn't work. I still hear voices. Every time I tell the doctors, they want to up my medication. I tell them, 'That will just make me angry,' because it will change the way I feel. Every time I tell them what's causing my problems, they say it's just my illness. It's not my illness" (field notes). Similarly, Carrie, a case management worker at Urban, tried to convince a client to take his medication as prescribed during his appointment with a psychiatric nurse. She said it was important for him to take his medication, because he'd had problems in the past when he had not done so. He could become violent and might have to go to the hospital. He could become threatening to staff. She said he was not like that when he was properly medicated. She said, "You might not see it, but others see it in you" (field notes).

Less commonly, expertise appeared grounded in the worker's status as a higher functioning and more competent individual in society than clients (as opposed to the clients' official status as lower-functioning and less competent).

This claim of expertise was especially called upon by workers without advanced clinical credentials. For instance, both Urban and Suburban offered staff-led computer groups for their clients. Suburban offered a computer group led by a worker with a high school degree (pursuing a bachelor's degree in the arts) with no special experience or credentials in computers. Nevertheless, he was purported to be (and indeed truly appeared to be, in my observation) more "expert" than most clients in his classes.[1] The paired facts that clients were involved with the organization to receive services and staff members were there to provide them could be used (in lieu of other claims) to demonstrate staff expertise.

Types of Institutionalization

So what forces bring together the disparate educational and professional backgrounds of workers and institutionalize a unifying logic? First, in the state where this study took place, a detailed and thorough set of *regulations* dictated exactly who could provide which services in Medicaid-funded organizations like the ones I studied, and also defined the set of professional knowledge that governed official interactions with clients.[2] These state administrative rules grouped a disparate array of professionals and paraprofessionals together into a hierarchy. At the top of the hierarchy was the LPHA (Licensed Practitioner of the Healing Arts), who could be a physician, nurse, psychologist, social worker, or counselor. The assumption was that these individuals possessed the proper certification, licensure, or experience to assess, diagnose, and recommend treatment for mental illness. Next came the QMHP (Qualified Mental Health Professional), with very similar but slightly less stringent qualifications than those required for the LPHA; it required less education (such as that of vocational counselors and RNs) and did not in all cases require licensing. Next came the MHP (Mental Health Professional), which required less education still—a bachelor's degree or extensive experience working in the mental health field (five years for those without a high school diploma). However, these individuals had to (in their past experience as well as in the current context) be supervised by a QMHP. Finally, there was the RSA (Rehabilitative Services Associate), which required only demonstrating "skills" for working in the mental health field. For each step in the hierarchy, those who met the qualifications of a given notch automatically met all of the requirements for those positions below them.

Being located in a given slot in this hierarchy meant that a worker could perform certain functions in the organization, formalizing jurisdiction and expertise. For instance, "Qs" and "Ls," as they were referred to around the agencies, had to sign off on certain paperwork, such as mental health assessments, for them to be valid—their expertise was determined necessary. The organizations billed the state at different rates for people in different positions doing the same service, formalizing that being higher in the hierarchy was more valuable. For instance, "client-centered consultation" performed by an RSA was billed at roughly 80 percent the rate of what it was billed if it was performed by an MHP.

In addition to crystallizing a value premium on education and licensing, however, these rules also institutionalized a body of expert knowledge as the driving force in dealing with client problems: psychotherapeutic knowledge. For instance, a diagnosis and assessment of functioning pulled from the American Psychiatric Association's *Diagnostic and Statistical Manual of Mental Disorders* was required for a prospective client to receive Medicaid-funded services. Though the psychologists, social workers, or counselors might differ somewhat in their orientations to mental health care, they all had sufficient education or experience to converse in therapeutic terms regarding clients.

There was another way jurisdiction and expertise was formalized through regulative institutionalization. Service definitions for different Medicaid-reimbursable services had guidelines for the professional backgrounds of who could provide the services. These were based not only on hierarchy, but also on profession. For instance, assertive community treatment (ACT) teams had to include a registered nurse and be in consultation with a psychiatrist, in addition to having at least one licensed clinician. The different domains of the lives of those receiving these services (such as mental health, physical health, income, and housing) were to be addressed by workers from distinct backgrounds.

In addition to regulation, however, there was also a *normative* component to this logic's institutionalization. This could be seen most starkly regarding expertise. In situations where some workers did not have professional credentials or a psychotherapeutic knowledge base, it was seen as a taboo or moral failing on the part of the worker, or on the organization for hiring the worker. Staff who themselves lacked the credentials and knowledge at times expressed a feeling of deficiency. One worker at Suburban without a college degree described it as follows: "I feel my deficiencies very, very keenly . . . in terms of, you know, education. I mean everybody that's here is, you know, geared up educationally to do this kind of work. They've, you know, got degrees in psychology . . . [or are] pursuing their master's in that same sort of thing. Um, and so—there are, you know, real basic fundamental kinds of things for them, that I don't even think of. . . . In some ways I'm even kind of, you know, surprised that they hired me" (interview). Those who lacked advanced education and training both judged themselves and at times felt judged by others as lacking in expertise and, thus, legitimacy.

Similar to the way state policy institutionalized a hierarchy of credentials, workers with psychotherapeutic credentials and knowledge might judge negatively those above them who lacked psychotherapeutic credentials or knowledge. For example, when I asked a worker at Suburban—who himself had a master's degree in counseling—about a former supervisor who I had heard had a tense relationship with staff, he responded with the following: "Let me just say that I am extremely happy with the current supervisors and their experience and educational credentials to back it up, and I am extremely confident in their ability to do their job effectively. Does that tell you anything?" (field notes). Another worker on an ACT team that was without an assigned clinical supervisor for much of my time there expressed what having a clinical supervisor would bring to her work experience: "Well, I mean, just meaning to your work" (interview). Without the viewpoint of a clinical expert, this staff member's daily work was at risk of being meaningless. Through both regulative and normative means, the clinical professional logic was institutionalized at Urban and Suburban.

The Empowerment Logic

There is no doubt that empowerment is a buzzword, and has been for decades. *The American Heritage Dictionary* notes that contemporary use of the word "empower" is rooted in the civil rights movement and women's movement of the 1960s, though it has diffused through society to be used by "people of all political persuasions" (Houghton Mifflin Company 2000:586). Its diffusion includes adoption by activists and advocates for people with mental illness (P. Brown 1981; McLean 2000). Although at least some elements of the logic could be found in the mental health care field before the 1960s (Dobransky 2009; Linhorst 2006), that is the decade when explicit calls for patient "empowerment" took off (Grob 1991). A major part of this spread was an incorporation of market mechanisms into the debate; most notable for the discussion here was a reconceptualization of members of disadvantaged groups as "consumers" of services who could demand to be heard (Cohen 2003). As a result, today you have "mental health consumers" (along with their families) advocating for themselves (McLean 2010).

At base, the empowerment logic says, from the patients' perspective, "Thanks, professionals, . . . [but] we don't think you as professionals can do it *for* us," as one movement leader said at a conference I attended with clients from

Suburban. He said that excluding clients from their treatment decision-making creates more stigma. "We can talk for ourselves," he said (field notes). Professionals, payers, and governmental entities all found rhetorical utility in the concept of client empowerment. However, there has been a great deal of ambiguity about how the concept is best translated into actual mental health practice (Dobransky 2009), and the devil is in those details. For instance, some mental health professionals argue that client competence is a prerequisite for client participation in services (Linhorst and Eckert 2003)—and determining competence is a professional task. Thus involving clients in treatment decision-making at the wrong time can oftentimes be *dis*-empowering (Peyser 2001; Zdanowicz 2006).

What is true for the broader empowerment logic is also true for the major treatment ideologies through which the logic has been brought into behavioral health services in the organizations I studied: "recovery" and "harm reduction" are inherently ambiguous concepts, though they are championed by Suburban and Urban, respectively. Recovery is problematized in that it can mean a reduction in symptoms ("recovery *from* mental illness") or a client-determined improvement in quality of life despite any level of symptoms ("recovery *in* mental illness") (Bellack 2006; Davidson and Roe 2007; Ralph 2005). Harm reduction is ambiguous when discussing who determines which harms to focus on and how to reduce those harms (Hall 2007; Obot 2007). Despite this ambiguity, the dominant interpretations of the empowerment logic and both treatment ideologies have a common central thread: *clients should be incorporated into treatment and organizational decision-making, both in the goals of treatment and in the means to achieve those goals.* Further, this ambiguity has not prevented the empowerment logic (and the empowerment-focused treatment ideologies) from being institutionalized in the mental health services system. Instead, it has led to a particular form of institutionalization.

Main Components

A central component of the empowerment logic at Urban and Suburban was *client self-determination* in the goals and modes of treatment. Though there were difficulties in truly carrying out this component of the logic in practice, it did happen. Perhaps the clearest ideal of how it could be done came from Flint, a manager at Urban, who discussed a hypothetical interaction with a client that solicited and respected the client's self-determination:

[*Client*]:   Man, I need to find a new place to live.
[*Worker*]: Well, what have you tried so far?

[*Client*]:   Well, I've tried A, B, and C.

[*Worker*]: Okay, and how's that going for you?

[*Client*]:   Not so well.

[*Worker*]: Well, what do you know that other people have tried?

[*Client*]:   Well, D, E, and F.

[*Worker*]: Okay, great. Why don't we think about that?

[*Client*]:   Okay, great.

[*Worker*]: So we've come up with A through F. Would it be okay if I may have some suggestions about G, H, and I, or, What would you think about that?

[*Client*]:   Yeah, sure man, I'll take whatever I can get.

[*Worker*]: Okay, here's G, H, I.

[*Client*]:   Oh, okay, well I hadn't thought about that.

[*Worker*]: Well, how can I help you with any of these? Do you want me to help you with any of these?

[*Client*]:   Yeah, I need your help.

[*Worker*]: Great, well then let's go and get this done. . . .

[*Client*]:   I spent—I spent my whole check up on cocaine again this month.

[*Worker*]: Okay, well what's that like for you, what happened?

[*Client*]:   Oh, I don't know if I can do it anymore. I need you to budget my money.

[*Worker*]: Well, what have you tried? [and so on]. . . .

> And I—I know it never works like this. But, you know, we do our best to solicit, to listen to whatever what have they done that's worked, what they thought about doing and then, with their permission, offer our suggestions, and then together come up with a plan to implement, and say, "Okay here's what you're going to do, here's what I'm gonna do, and here's how we're gonna know if it's working" (interview).

With perhaps a more practical bent, Marin, a manager at Suburban, found that many of the problems that present themselves to him as a supervisor in the organization arise from the workers "getting ahead" of the clients:

> Well, the major pattern that would be true for all of us is that, you know, we want change when a person is not ready for change. We [feel we] know what's best for the person, and I would not even [say] that we're wrong [about feeling that]. . . . But the mistake we make over and over is our wanting it doesn't make it so. . . . And actually, it might interfere with, you know, helping a client to make it so. . . . [Sometimes I have

to help workers] see where they might be blocking the change by wanting it more than the client, you know. Sometimes backing away allows
the person to move forward, when you're the person in the way, at least
metaphorically. . . . You can't change people and it's even very hard to
lead them to change. (interview)

So, although the ideal may not be realized, there is a push to allow clients to
change at their own pace and to make their own decisions when possible.

Another major component of the empowerment logic was to work with
the client to *remove barriers* that lie in the way of their reaching goals and to
help clients *obtain resources* to reach goals. A good deal of mental health services is focused on dealing with barriers internal to the client. So, for example,
symptoms may interfere with the client acting in a constructive and functional
way (Linhorst and Eckert 2003), so medication management and helping clients develop skills and psychotherapeutic resources to deal with symptoms
when they arise are major parts of casework. In addition, people with chronic
mental illness and those who have been homeless for long periods often lack
basic living skills such as money management, hygiene, and social skills, defi-
cits that may stand in the way of other goals a client may have, such as securing
and maintaining independent housing or employment (Schutt and Goldfinger
2011). Thus, staff worked with clients on these internal barriers.

In addition to internal barriers, the staff at both organizations worked
to help clients address external barriers. These external barriers were wide-
ranging, located at the local, state, and national levels. For instance, staff at both
organizations advocated for clients with local landlords or other residential
facilities who might not want to provide housing to them. As Urban's clients'
drug and alcohol issues often put them in contact with law enforcement, staff
advocated for them in court hearings as well. In addition, Urban affiliated with
local political advocacy organizations to try to change drug laws to reduce their
negative impact on clients. Along with legal aid, they also helped clients obtain
benefits from Social Security. Staff at Suburban worked as mediators with local
businesses to help clients overcome barriers to employment. Suburban (with
some other local organizations) also held meetings and debates featuring local
state government officials and candidates to focus attention on mental health
policy and funding. By carrying out this range of advocacy activities, staff
worked to connect clients to resources they otherwise might not have access to.
The two organizations also organized and participated with clients in rallies at
the state capitol to protect state funding for mental health services. This worked
to maintain resources not only for clients, but also for staff themselves.

A final component of the empowerment logic evident at both organizations was *peer support*. A concerted effort was made at both organizations to connect clients with other current and former clients who had experienced success in dealing with the same problems that clients faced. The belief was that these individuals, serving as people who truly understood what clients were going through because they went (or were still going) through it themselves, could, in the words of the twelve-step movement, "share experience, strength, and hope" with the clients. They provided a model for change that professionals without such a background could not (Clay et al. 2005; A. Scott 2012). There were a few ways the organizations did this. First, both hired "prosumers," people who had themselves dealt with the issues confronting clients and were working to help others: at Suburban, the issue was primarily mental illness; at Urban, it could be mental illness, substance abuse, homelessness, or prison. Suburban had what it called an "affirmative" hiring policy for people with mental illness, giving them preferential consideration. At both organizations, prosumer positions were often distinct from other positions in that the individual was part-time at an RSA position—in part to avoid losing any government benefits the employees may receive, but also to avoid overstressing the employee. However, as these workers gained experience (at least five years, by state regulation, unless they possessed clinical credentials), they sometimes moved into full-time MHP positions.

In addition to having prosumers as employees, Suburban's parent organization, Wellness, also had clients (including some at Suburban) who were not employees serve in leadership positions. Wellness used a nationally recognized client leadership and self-advocacy curriculum to try to cultivate leaders among clients. Suburban also had elected positions on its client council. Non-employee clients also led groups at Suburban. In these cases, a staff member usually consulted with the client leader and sat in the group. However, at the behest of the client recovery administrator at Wellness, there was a short-lived peer support group that met without any involvement by Suburban's staff (though the administrator was herself involved when the group started and the group petered out shortly after she stopped attending).

Types of Institutionalization

The empowerment logic was most strongly institutionalized *normatively*. There has been widespread endorsement of client self-determination throughout the mental health system. The rhetorical force of such claims is hard to miss and can be found at all levels of the system. For instance, the influential report of the President's New Freedom Commission on Mental Health held as one of its key goals for the future of the mental health system that services should be "consumer- and family-driven" and care should be "consumer-centered, with providers working in full partnership with the consumers they serve" (President's New Freedom Commission on Mental Health 2003:27–28). As a presidential commission, however, the document is not binding policy. A similar state-level document gave a "vision" of recovery that viewed successful outcomes in a recovery-oriented state mental health system in part through clients acting on their right to make independent choices regarding their own community engagement and personal, social, monetary, or vocational goals. Again, however, this is a vision statement, not binding regulation.

Unlike the application of the empowerment logic to people with mental illness, however, when the client population consisted of substance abusers (with or without other mental illnesses), normative institutionalization was not evident at the level of policy. This can be seen during 2005 testimony before a US House Subcommittee that was provocatively titled "Harm Reduction or Harm Maintenance?: Is There Such a Thing as Safe Drug Abuse?" (United States Congress House Committee 2005). Advocates of harm reduction at the hearing argued it was a humane and practical approach to reducing the negative impact of drug use, and sound public health policy, akin to speed limits and seatbelts. However, opponents of harm reduction at the hearing claimed that, even if the term had once referred to legitimate treatment (which they doubted), it had been "hijacked" by drug legalization advocates. Moreover, they claimed that allowing clients to continue engaging in active drug use actually maintained the harm of drug addiction. Even though support for the treatment ideology might not be widespread, there was a segment of the behavioral health services sector that strongly supported and promoted it. Urban was affiliated with this segment. It is important to note, though, that clients at Urban with drug problems were dually diagnosed with both substance use disorders and severe mental illness. Therefore, by focusing on the mental illness side of the diagnosis, Urban could shield itself from some of the negative reactions provoked by endorsing self-determination for its clients. Some elements of the harm reduction approach to treatment—such as motivational interviewing—were even considered legitimate, evidence-based practices in the mental health care sector (Drake et al. 2001a).

An important accrediting body for both Urban and Suburban was the Commission on the Accreditation of Rehabilitation Facilities, or CARF. This accreditation supplied legitimacy for those providing services to people with chronic mental illness. Accrediting organizations such as these are enormously important for normative institutionalization at the field level (W. Scott 2008; W. Scott et al. 2000). On a section of its website aimed at prospective clients of its accredited facilities, the organization claimed to ensure true consumer participation in organizational operation:

> Choosing CARF-accredited programs and services gives you the assurance that:
>
> - The programs or services actively involve consumers in selecting, planning, and using services.
> - The organization's programs and services have met consumer-focused, state-of-the-art international standards of performance.
> - These standards were developed with the involvement and input of consumers.
> - The organization is focused on assisting each consumer in achieving his or her chosen goals and outcomes.[3]

CARF standards manuals included sections titled "Input from Stakeholders," "Rights of Persons Served," and "Individual-Centered Service Planning, Design, and Delivery," each including criteria with which organizations had to demonstrate compliance. Guidelines stated that organizations must show that they provided clients with information and sought client input both on the clients' own treatment and on organizational operation. Audits for reaccreditation occurred every few years. Thus, unlike state-level rhetoric, CARF rhetoric had some teeth behind it.

Moving from the field level to daily life inside Urban and Suburban, normative institutionalization was once again evident. For instance, when I first introduced myself to clients at Suburban, I mentioned the word "rehabilitation" as part of the goal of the organization. A vocal client named Daniel quickly spoke up and said, "We don't do rehabilitation here; we do recovery" (field notes). In staff meetings as well, "recovery" was imposed as the appropriate orientation for workers, usually emphasizing the importance of respecting client self-determination. At one representative meeting, for instance, staff discussed a party organized by clients, and the issue of the food that would be served was raised. One of the client organizers wanted to have pizza. A staff member said that she "told [the client] no. It's going to be at 2 P.M. in the afternoon, you're not having pizza." A supervisor immediately prompts the worker, tacking on "in the most recovery-oriented way possible." The implication here was that the worker's statement was directive. The supervisor's statement raised (somewhat awkwardly) the recovery ideology to point out that fact and implied that workers should watch such language and behavior—or at least reconsider bringing it up in the meeting in my presence. The same supervisor did the exact same thing to another worker later in the meeting (field notes). This sort of interaction happened routinely. Even though staff often expressed not having a clear idea of what recovery meant, the general concern with client self-determination was clear.

The same type of normative pressure was also at work regarding harm reduction at Urban. Regularly, even in the most extreme circumstances, the treatment ideology was introduced as an organizing point in conversations regarding clients. This is illustrated by staff's discussion of conflict between two clients in the day program. One of the clients had brought in a weapon for self-protection, and it was inadvertently publicly displayed. A major conflict between that client, the other client, and staff ensued. In discussing the issue later at a staff meeting, workers considered whether to let the client who brought the weapon continue to attend the program. Some workers said that if the client had turned the weapon in to staff when he came to the program and retrieved it when he left, it would not have been a problem. Two workers say—in unison—that checking of weapons was acceptable "with harm reduction" (meaning within the harm reduction approach to service delivery) (field notes).

Those who did not strongly support harm reduction nonetheless felt its normative embeddedness in the program, as was evident one day when I was observing a group of workers discussing Involvement, a harm-reduction-focused program at Urban that had closed when its grant funding ran out. Many of its workers had diffused throughout Urban's other programs, including those I studied. On this particular occasion, none of those former employees were present. After one worker mentioned Involvement by name, another sarcastically said "you forgot to make the sign of the cross" when saying the program's name. I asked about that, and they said some workers and administrators at Urban thought it was the end-all-be-all of services. I ask what they thought about it. One worker said that it was "very good at doing the liberal end of the harm reduction model. If that was its goal, then it was effective" (field notes).

In addition to this normative institutionalization, workers at both organizations experienced the empowerment logic through its *regulative* institutionalization, as well, though more weakly than with the clinical-professional logic. There were some concrete legal decisions regarding respecting clients' rights and preferences, such as the US Supreme Court's *Olmstead v. L.C.* decision, which stated mental health clients cannot be kept in state hospitals against their will if it is determined they could adequately be treated in community settings.

However, these regulations were never brought up in the organizations. Other policies were a bit less concrete and, I would argue, more symbolic. After the President's New Freedom Commission report was released, many states worked to implement its consumer-focused goal. In a follow-up document, titled *Trends in Mental Health System Transformation: The States Respond* (2006), the federal government's Substance Abuse and Mental Health Services Administration lauded the efforts of states in moving toward the goal. Though somewhat vague, the report notes that some states adopted "person-centered planning"—explicitly involving clients in treatment decision-making—as well as funding consumer-run services and having consumers serve on state mental health planning councils. The federal government requires states receiving funding to have consumer representation on state mental health councils (McLean 2000). Still, some states ran into difficulties implementing the empowerment logic in policy. Jacobson (2004) highlights some of the problems Wisconsin had in putting the recovery ideology into practice. She explains that part of the issue was the lack of clarity about the definition of "recovery," and another issue was that the state was concurrently implementing managed behavioral health care, which conflicted with some of what were thought to be recovery-focused policy orientations. In the state where my research was conducted, a "vision statement" for public mental health services published around the time my research began explicitly noted that state-level funding was lacking for recovery-oriented services. Further, although some federal government grants (some of which Urban had secured) might fund harm-reduction-focused programs for a limited time, ongoing funding was quite precarious.

In addition to its role in normative institutionalization, CARF accreditation led to some of the most concrete regulative institutionalization of the empowerment logic at Urban and Suburban. One reason for this was that state policy used accreditation to forgo its own auditing of organizations. If mental health care sites were accredited by organizations such as CARF, the state assumed they were complying with a host of state regulations. Because CARF had concrete standards for client involvement, the state, by proxy, could be seen as enforcing these as regulations. One CARF requirement was that each organization "demonstrates" that it "obtains input . . . on an ongoing basis . . . from . . . persons served." One suggested way of doing so was to have a client "advisory council," which both Urban and Suburban had. The council was a formal venue through which clients could raise concerns, ask questions, and have input into organizational operation. Both Urban and Suburban had a council, but each operated quite differently. Clients at Suburban actually elected formal officers for different positions within the council, and the council was frequently charged with formal decisions regarding client activities and, on occasion, with coming up with ideas to deal with organizational problems. Urban, on the other hand, ran their council like an informal information-dissemination and discussion forum.

A second CARF (and state) requirement that both organizations implemented was the personalized treatment plan (PTP).[4] With this document as a template, staff and the client were to work together to establish goals for the client to achieve with the help of the organization. The plans covered broad goals, specific objectives, and service interventions offered by the organizations to assist clients in achieving the goals. There were four broad areas covered by the plans: physical health, mental health, social integration/recovery, and alcohol and substance abuse. Not all clients had formal goals in all areas; Urban's plans were more structured than Suburban's and were more likely to include goals in each area. Given that Urban's clients were more often homeless and dually diagnosed with substance abuse and mental illness, this is understandable. There were scheduled reviews of the plans to make sure clients still agreed with the same goals and to measure progress toward goals. The period of review was generally every three or six months. In addition to these preplanned reviews, PTPs were supposed to be updated any time major transitions occurred in the client's life (for example, change in residence, admission to or discharge from the hospital or inpatient drug treatment) or when the client decided to change his or her goals.

Although the plans did exist at both organizations, workers detailed difficulties in truly incorporating clients in the treatment plan development for a couple of reasons. First, some workers said clients changed their goals frequently. For instance, Katy, a worker at Urban, described how this commonly occurred when reviewing treatment goals in PTPs with clients: "[Regarding substance abuse goals,] somebody may initially want to reduce their use. Then they may decide then to stop their use. They may go in the opposite direction [increasing use again]. They may decide [that substance abuse is] not what they want to work on. They [may instead] want to get a job. . . . You know what, that's awesome that they're doing that. But then I'm confused as a worker. I was like, 'Oh wait, I had all these like things organized in my head'" (interview). These frequent changes were difficult for workers to incorporate efficiently into the paperwork of the treatment plan and, more importantly, made it difficult for workers to develop consistent, sustained treatment interventions with clients. A second, perhaps more common issue was that workers described clients as very ambivalent or apathetic about setting clear goals to work toward. Life spent in "total institutions" or with family had left many clients very passive and dependent on staff to make decisions and set goals for them.

Finally, state Medicaid mental health service definitions led to the empowerment logic also being institutionalized through regulative means. If an organization provided ACT, their teams were required to have a mental health consumer on the team to receive state funding, formalizing the peer support component of the logic. Community support team service definitions recommended, but did not require, a consumer on the team. So, the empowerment logic was strongly institutionalized normatively, and less strongly through regulative means.

The Community Logic

Concerns with "community" have pervaded social thinkers and mental health care providers for over a century (Schutt and Goldfinger 2011). The roots of the community logic in mental health treatment can be traced to the late eighteenth and early nineteenth century and the rise of "moral treatment" and the asylum (Grob 1994; Morrissey and Goldman 1986; Shorter 1997). The core idea was that the social environment in which a patient resides can play a part in causing or treating mental illness, and that creating a more stable, healthy environment could thus eliminate mental illness. Unlike later incarnations, however, this early version of the community logic centered on isolating patients from society, not incorporating them into it.

Observation of the extreme effects of post-traumatic illness in soldiers returning from World War II provided renewed evidence that the social environment could greatly impact mental health. This later dovetailed with the passion for social change of the 1960s, yielding "the community mental health ideology" (Grob 1991). As formalized by Frank Baker and Herbert Schulberg (1967), the ideology saw mental health professionals as having responsibility for both acute treatment and public health, both of which should involve engagement in and with the community.

During the late 1970s, the focus shifted from the entire "community" population to people with severe, persistent mental illness. The needs of this population had been neglected in previous eras. However, as state mental hospitals emptied, the harsh realities of inadequate community-based services for released patients finally led to a strategy to address their needs: community support (Tessler and Goldman 1982; Turner and TenHoor 1978). Though originating in a federal National Institute of Mental Health–funded pilot program, the community support approach has since filtered down to become a dominant underlying logic at the state level, where community mental health services are largely managed today (Dill 2001; Floersch 2000). The ideology as originally outlined involves ten components, including the provision of services with no set end date to clients wherever they might be found. The services were not restricted to managing the clinical symptoms of illness, but also included basic social and financial supports. There was an explicit focus on partnering with community and family members and on protecting clients' rights. The overall goal of the program was to wrap clients in services that would allow them to maintain their health and quality of life outside of the hospital setting (Turner and TenHoor 1978).

Main Components

A major thrust of the community logic as experienced at Urban and Suburban was *integration with the "natural."* The assumption was that anything associated with the mental health organization was considered "artificial" or, as Elizabeth Townsend describes it, a "simulation" (Townsend 1998). Clients might obtain resources or learn coping or life skills in mental health care organizations, but these benefits might not transfer well to life outside the organization, which was where clients spent most of their time. As one manager at Urban said, "[E]ven if someone comes here [for the day program] for a full five hours and gets an ACT home visit, that's six. I mean that's six hours in their day, you know. There's eighteen more to go, so—and then the weekends, right?" (interview). Thus, a goal was to break down those barriers between organizational life and the rest of the clients' lives.

There were two parts to integration with the natural: providing services in clients' *natural setting* and building clients' *natural support.* First, if the same service could be provided in the mental health facility or the "community" outside it, then the latter was definitely preferable. Because a major component of both programs (especially Suburban) was a day program, the implementation of this aspect of the logic was limited in some ways (though Urban also had ACT/community support teams, which were much more community-engaged). Nevertheless, staff did go "out into the community" with clients. So, instead of simply talking with clients abstractly about how to take the bus, staff members at Suburban actually went with them to use the bus. A fitness group at Suburban combined exercise on the organization's equipment with trips to a local recreation center. Suburban also had a "community access" group in which clients did things such as learn how to use landmarks and directions when navigating a neighborhood. Various activity groups at Urban took clients to local businesses, museums, and parks. Case management workers from Urban also regularly met with clients in their own homes, and outreach workers went searching for prospective clients on the streets, in shelters, and at other places in the community where they might be found.

The second part of integration with the natural was that the organization was to work with the client to build natural supports. Although there is no doubt that the organizations were supposed to, in the short term, work as a support system for clients, the community logic dictates that dependence on the organization should be minimized in degree and duration (to the extent possible), with "the community" replacing the organization as the source of support. So, clients could be employed by Suburban at the sheltered workshop (a form of work demonstrating dependence on the facility), but the organization also had a successful vocational team that could find clients jobs (usually entry-level retail) outside the organization. Urban had a vocational worker for a time as well (before my research began), but the program was not continued when the worker left the organization. Much more common at Urban was case management workers helping clients to pursue Social Security disability benefits. In either case, having the added income could help clients obtain sources of financial support other than what the organization could provide them with directly.

According to the community logic, in addition to helping with financial support, organizations were to work with clients to build community-based social and emotional supports. Ideally, the various community activities in which both organizations involved clients could serve as models of the types of things clients would do on their own. At Suburban, the client recovery administrator also worked to connect clients with other peers in community-based peer support organizations. Several workers at Urban were themselves members of twelve-step self-help groups and referred clients to those groups. Helping clients manage or rekindle family relationships was another way workers could help clients build community-based supports. Although much less common at Urban, at Suburban some workers had regular contact with clients' families—in part because a number of clients lived with their families.

Another major component of the community logic, which had considerable overlap with integration with the natural, is that organizations worked to push clients toward *independence*—both independence in general and, especially, independence from the mental health system. In first engaging the client in services, temporary dependence was acceptable. However, the end goal of services was to push clients toward living and managing their affairs on their own to the degree possible, drastically reducing or eliminating organizational services when the client was deemed to no longer need or want them. Much interaction among workers regarding clients centered on whether clients were "ready" to take a step toward more independence. This discussion could be about whether a client who wanted to take a step had "progressed" enough to take the step, or it could be about whether a client who did not want to take the step should be pushed to do so. This process was evident during a staff meeting at Suburban in which staff discussed a client's interest in independent housing and community employment.

> Brandy brings up Phillip. He's been here for a year. She said this is the first time he's gone a year without going to the hospital. She said he hates [the nursing facility where he lives]. Brandy said she's [looking to] maybe get some independent housing for him. . . . Somebody suggests he [work in the workshop] so he can lay the groundwork for working [outside the facility]. . . . Brandy said his work history is "spotty." Brandy says he [worked in the workshop] before and he didn't like it. . . . Brandy said, "If he was close to getting housing, he would get a job." Monique says, "Housing takes time. He has to see it as 'paying my keep,' which is what it is." She says living on his own, he couldn't afford a doctor or a room. Brandy restates that she will work with [vocational] to get him a job if he's close to getting housing. Georgette said he needs to "get used to a job," or else he will "falter." Monique says he needs to "get used to paying out money." Glenda says, "He has to want to do it. But if he doesn't, that's what we have to go for [what he wants], and he may falter." (field notes)

Not all workers at this meeting were sure that the way Phillip and his worker wanted to move toward independence was the best way, but he seemed a good candidate for that move given his desire and his improving symptoms. Though much rarer at Urban, where much focus was on just trying to keep clients engaged with the organization, these pushes toward more independence did take place. For example, one worker, Taylor, tried to push a client, Ronde, to move out of the very small, run-down apartment he lived in, as he had a decent income and the worker thought he could afford a nicer apartment. On the way to meet with Ronde, Taylor told me he thought Ronde should try to get a larger, nicer place, because he has the money. However, Ronde was content where he was and had told Taylor so repeatedly. Taylor stated that such reservations could be another "negative symptom" of schizophrenia. Taylor said they had him ready to move at one point, but with some organizational changes taking place, management did not want to add that to the list of changes. When Taylor met with Ronde, the client said he had been working out at the local park gym three times a week and looking at the Internet at a local place that charged a dollar an hour. Taylor suggested he may want to move out, using a jocular manner that minimized threat or judging. Ronde replied, as usual, that he was happy where he was. Taylor persisted, saying, "You can afford it." On the walk out of the building, Taylor was a little more toned down, bringing it up again. "I know we talk about that a lot. You deserve a bigger place" (field notes). Ronde had clearly taken steps toward independence, but Taylor thought there was one more he could take, and pushed him to do so.

Types of Institutionalization

Since the late 1970s, the community logic has been strongly institutionalized through the *regulative* dimension. In case law, the Supreme Court's *Olmstead* decision cemented a client's right to community-based settings if the client wanted that placement and if he or she could be adequately treated there. Further, community support, ACT, and psychosocial rehabilitation (PSR), three key services geared toward community integration that both organizations provided, were Medicaid-billable at the state level. PSR was generally provided within the facility, but offered skills training for clients to prepare them for community life. The other two services focused on providing services outside the facility. Community support services were considered less intensive (for instance, requiring less frequent visits with clients) than ACT and were reimbursed for less money; however, they were practically the same services. Taken together, the services were geared toward providing clients with tools and resources that would eventually lead to independence from the mental health system to the degree possible.

Changes to state mental health policy, in the state where my research occurred, shared an underlying theme: to move clients with severe mental illness, over time, from the physical organizations themselves to the surrounding community. Lower functioning clients and those with more severe symptoms could still receive services at the organizations, but as they stabilized, there was a push—both in services available and in funding—to move them into "the community." Under the state community support service definition, combined community support services provided by any organization seeking reimbursement from the state must take place in clients' "natural setting" (which policy assumes is outside of mental health services facilities) a minimum of 60 percent of the time. These state policies were enforced by regular audits of organizational operation.

After new policy was adopted during my research, both organizations moved a large portion of their services to community support. At a meeting at Urban explaining the changed state service definitions to workers, an administrator made the message from the state very clear: they preferred the organization to provide services in the community instead of in the organization—community support services instead of "creating chronic PSR clients" (field notes). A manager at Suburban said that this was going to lead mental health care providers to "get rid of the real estate," as there would be fewer services taking place at facilities—there would be more "roaming workers" (field notes).

In the past, this regulative institutionalization was accompanied by a strong normative type as well, with moral reformers arguing against keeping mental patients locked in hospitals. However, during my research, I found this less the case. Instead, the underlying thrust of the logic was firmly entrenched in workers' minds. It was assumed that movement to the community, to whatever degree, was the ultimate goal for clients. As opposed to a consciously articulated and symbolically loaded endorsement (that is, a *normative* institutionalization), staff at both Urban and Suburban acted on a unified but never fully articulated vision of the community logic—a *cultural-cognitive* institutionalization.

The vision starts with the view that some people are in dire need of mental health services and do not receive them. Those people need to be located and "engaged" with the mental health system, receiving the services they need. Once they receive those services, are stabilized, and make "progress," learning the skills they need to be functional in the "natural" community outside the organization, they can "graduate" from an intensive service provider and move on. The next destination could be a provider of less intensive services or full-fledged independent living. Though staff at both organizations held this vision, Urban and Suburban considered themselves at different points within the vision's model. Because of Urban's clientele—homeless, with severe co-occurring substance abuse and mental illness problems, and many with limited engagement with services—the organization often functioned as the link between disengaged clients and their first sustained contact with services. Suburban, on the other hand, with its clientele more stable in housing and symptoms, generally served as the means for clients to move from higher-intensity services to less intensive services or to independence. Further, though staff institutionalized this vision through cultural-cognitive means, not all staff agreed on how it should be applied in any particular circumstance. So, for instance, although independent living was the ultimate goal for clients, the relative "readiness" of any individual client to make that move could be (and was) debated among staff.

Both organizations had at one time or another formally implemented this vision in their structure of services. For a time, Urban had subdivided services based on perceived client function and need, with clients progressing to different "teams" within the organization, each with distinct expectations and intensity of services. At some point clients could "graduate" out of the organization to a less intensive service provider. However, Urban decided to eliminate that structure before my research began. Suburban did not formally divide services, but they did have rituals and formal evaluation of progress through their program. When a client "passed" enough groups and achieved other benchmarks, they would "move up a level," eventually reaching "graduation," where they were seen as making maximum "progress" through the program. There were annual ceremonies for clients moving up levels and for graduations. In addition to (or perhaps underlying) the formal structures, however, staff at both organizations held the community logic in their minds. I found discussions of these issues common at both organizations, regardless of the formal structure. Note that the discussions were about where to place individual clients on the spectrum of the community logic, not discussions questioning the vision itself.

Cultural-cognitive institutionalization is difficult to detect in research settings because elements are rarely explicitly stated (Schneiberg and Clemens 2006). However, I found that the vision could be detected, in pieces and parts, in staff's interactions with each other and with clients and through pressing staff to articulate their positions during interviews. One way it was detectable was through its serving as a basis for elaboration. When staff explained why a course of action was appropriate, they cited aspects of the vision, reminding everyone of their shared conceptions of what they do. Occasionally, when discussing clients during meetings and conversations with each other, staff stated part of the vision as a jumping-off point to argue for some particular strategy. For instance, in one meeting at Suburban, staff discussed how to handle a client in the group home who was several months behind paying rent, but who had not yet been kicked out. One worker, Monique, asked "How does that prepare him for the real world if there are no consequences. In the real world—if he was on his own, he would be put out on the street" (field notes). The implication was that preparing clients for the "real world"—independence—was what the organization was supposed to do. Similarly, at a staff meeting at Urban, a worker was concerned about beds left open at a housing unit, and how that related to Urban's role in the community logic. There was an issue with some of the beds in one of the housing units, with discussion of how long to hold the beds. Both the business director, who was not present, and Bobby, a worker who was present, wanted them to get filled more quickly. Bobby said that their goal was to connect people with services, and having beds open while people are on the street was a problem. Someone pointed out that they had to do some paperwork before they could house the client. Bobby replied that they should move that along (field notes). Again we see a worker explicitly stating what is rarely articulated—a shared understanding (which was not challenged) of the organization's placement on the community logic's spectrum.

Logic of Bureaucratic Accountability

In tracing the major institutional eras in US health care since the middle of the twentieth century, Peter Mendel, W. Richard Scott, and colleagues describe a progression, from a time when the medical profession dominated through periods when first the government and then corporate and standard-setting bodies joined the increasingly crowded field. A major theme running through these changes is that a growing number of actors wanted to control various aspects of the delivery of health care, especially cost and quality (Mendel and Scott 2010; Scott et al. 2000). Institutional changes like these in the broader health care arena "spill over" into the mental health services system, for which they are, perhaps, less well suited (Schlesinger and Gray 1999).

A range of actors is attempting to influence the delivery of care in the present era. Some appear to be unified by a desire to hold providers and recipients of care accountable, and to base that accountability on the bureaucratic tracking, documentation, and auditing of service provision (cf. Casalino 2004). Tapping into an increasing distrust of professionals throughout society (Freidson 2001), these actors attempt to undercut decoupling between standards and practice (Hallett 2010), trying to structure care to address the priorities they hold dear, such as cost-containment, efficiency, industry standards, consumer rights, and scientific evidence. Similar changes have been found in education (Hallett 2010) and law (Espeland and Vannebo 2007).

Within the health care field, some of the central concerns regarding quality in this movement toward bureaucratic accountability are well represented by a 2001 report by the Institute of Medicine (IOM), *Crossing the Quality Chasm*. The report highlighted a major gap between advancements in science on one hand and the implementation of these advancements in health care practice on the other. Among other improvements in the health care system, the report recommended the following:

> All health care organizations, professional groups, private and pub-lic purchasers should pursue six major aims; specifically, health care should be safe, effective, patient-centered, timely, efficient, and equi-table. . . . Congress should continue to authorize and appropriate funds for, and the Department of Health and Human services should move for-ward expeditiously with the establishment of, monitoring and tracking process for use in evaluating the progress of the health system in pursuit of the above cited aims. (Institute of Medicine 2001:6–7)

In a 2006 follow-up report, the IOM argues that, although there are some differences between general health care and behavioral health services in the United States, "the *Quality Chasm* framework can be applied to health care for mental and substance use conditions" (Institute of Medicine 2006:2). Among other recommendations, the report says that government funders in mental health services should cut back on grant-based funding mechanisms and tie funding to quality performance measures. It also argues for prioritizing funding for evidence-based practices—an increasing trend in health care more broadly (Timmermans 2010; Timmermans and Berg 2003)—while acknowledging that the evidence base is not as strong in mental health and addiction services as it is in general health care.

Alongside this move to improve the measurement of quality in behavioral health care has been a push by both the public and the private sectors to contain costs in mental health services.[5] Though the full-fledged dominance of man-aged care organizations in the health care sector was never attained, the broader concern in both public and private health care—including mental health care—with using various mechanisms to contain costs has persisted (Mechanic 2004; Scheid 2003; Scheid 2004). As Teresa Scheid states, in the move to contain costs, the distinction between the public and the private sectors is "becom-ing blurred" (Scheid 2004:6). States are using private health care management companies to revamp and contain costs in their Medicaid systems, including in behavioral health (Mechanic 2007).

These concerns for cost and quality are two major targets of bureaucratic accountability in mental health care, but what is central to the logic is less the content of what is tracked than it is the drive for measurement, documentation, and oversight itself, as well as the lack of trust in professional and organizational self-governance.

Main Components

It was impossible to be a worker at either organization and successfully avoid *documentation*. So essential was the formal logging of workers' activities that a documentation "best practices" manual from Suburban stated outright, "NOTH-ING I have done today in my job happened, [*sic*] until I document it." Every interaction workers had with or about clients had to at least be considered for documentation. Further, that documentation should correspond to goals and objectives in the client's personalized treatment plan. If the event did not strictly appear to qualify, workers might have to alter aspects of the event to make it fit documentation standards. As one worker at Suburban said, if someone has "an eight-minute conversation [with a client] with no substance," the worker has to "make stuff up." The worker noted that management told staff not to make things up, but some clients say "the same thing ten times a day," which made fabrication hard to avoid (field notes). The documentation requirements could wear on workers. "Every time I have a conversation with someone, I have an hour of paperwork [because of it]," one worker at Urban lamented (field notes).

A good portion of what workers documented were the activities of their clients. From the moment they first interacted with an outreach worker until they said their last good-byes, clients were subject to constant monitoring and documenting. With policy and documentation software changes, this tendency only increased. For example, in addition to entering individual notes about each client in each group, workers at Suburban also had to note if clients arrived to groups late, left early, or left and came back. Several workers found the requirement extremely problematic, because some clients left and reentered groups several times. Clients often had to sign in and sign out of different locations to document they were there. This could present problems for clients who did not sign (intentionally or accidentally) or who were illiterate. Because it was important to have their presence documented, staff would, on occasion, fill in a client's name on the client's behalf. One day at Urban, a worker, Steve, was doing so; a client named Lonnie became angry and had to have the importance of signing in explained to him by another worker:

> Steve and Cindy talk about who is going to take which participants on their respective sign-in sheets . . . Lonnie yells over to Steve [even though he is close], "Steve, don't you sign my name on that sheet." Steve responds with "Lonnie, I'm not going to have this conversation." Lonnie

repeats his statement louder, and Steve repeats his in the same low tone. Lonnie finally yells again, "Don't you sign my name on that sheet if I'm not going to a group!" Steve says, "Let's go out in the hall." They go out in the hall. They come back in. . . . Ariana's involved after that. I see her across the room, and I can hear her saying to Lonnie that in order to be [in the day program], he has to have his name on the sheet. (field notes)

Lonnie appeared not to understand that his presence in the common area during lunchtime was billed as being in a group. Similarly, at Suburban, early in my research, time that clients were not in a group was referred to as "milieu" time. Though workers themselves did not have to create documentation about that time, it was documented (and billed for) by the organization's administrative staff and software. Later in my research, things changed and the only time that was documented and billed was time that workers actually interacted with or about clients (which they had to document), which again increased the amount of documentation for workers.

One of the main reasons the documentation was important was that auditors might examine it; it had to conform to the standards of those who processed and checked the documentation. This could lead to straying from "accurately" portraying an event. For instance, at a staff meeting at Suburban, there was a discussion of how they entered service notes into the system. An example given on a handout was what appeared to be a very detailed note of a clinical interaction with a client involving concerns she had "about her son, her medications, her resume, and her trust issues with people." However, the critique from the administrative department was that there was too much detail, especially about medications, and that the interaction was not packaged clearly enough for the service it was listed under—counseling. An "alternative format" was distributed that was a third the length of the original note and tailored much more to counseling. A manager said, "The only way to get over this hurdle is to be vague, broad, and all-encompassing. . . . Clarity works against us." In order to meet the requirements of various possible auditors, prepackaged options and language were distributed in "best practices" manuals, and some were built into documentation software. So, it should come as no surprise that a manager said in that same meeting (of the alternative format), "You can see that you could easily copy and paste this, changing a few things for any meeting you have with a client" (field notes). I likewise saw workers at Urban creating documents with "standard phrasing" that they could then copy and paste into service notes.

Another major component of the logic of bureaucratic accountability at Urban and Suburban was *standardization*. One of the first things I was told when my research at Suburban began was that its parent organization, Wellness, under new leadership, was trying to unify the services and practices of all the different programs within the organization. The previous leadership had allowed programs such as Suburban to be more creative and "entrepreneurial" in their approaches, and to try new things. New leadership valued consistency more, so that a client could go to any program and know what to expect. Although workers were perhaps less conscious of or vocal about it, aspects of the trend were also evident at Urban. CARF accreditation was a major standardizing force, requiring both organizations to adopt a range of practices and procedures. Numerous times throughout my research I heard staff members say that they were engaging in some practice because it was "required by CARF" or because "CARF says we have to do it."

Urban and Suburban incorporated many evidence-based practices—interventions with set protocols and guidelines—in their programs. At Urban, assertive community treatment was a major component of the program early on. However, with changes in state policy, the organization chose to abandon the service and instead shift all existing ACT clients to the new community support service. A manager explained to me that, though the organization had considered keeping one ACT team for the most severely ill, the new state service definitions were too strict to make implementation realistic. "The thirty-first consecutive day that that team was down [a] staff person [the organization] can no longer bill ACT services" (interview). The organization could bill for community support services for that team's work—but only after the client treatment plans were changed to reflect the shift from ACT to community support. Although the manager seemed to view this as a cost-saving measure by the state ("the state, like, intentionally redefined ACT services in a way that nobody would want—would be able to afford to run an ACT program" [interview]), another way to view it is that the state intentionally tied funding to "fidelity" to the ACT model.

Another evidence-based practice that Urban used was dialectical behavioral therapy (DBT). The program combined group treatment with individual therapy. Staff said it was implemented in response to client demand for more involved services once progress was made on meeting their basic needs. However, over the course of my research, it became apparent that clients were not willing or able to maintain the level of involvement or commitment necessary to participate in the formalized program. Thus, the organization implemented what they called "DBT-Light," which meant they kept the groups (without strict attendance requirements) and tried to engage willing participants in individual therapy as well. Although Urban made an effort, the realities of the client population and funding prevented the implementation of evidence-based practices in ways that closely adhered to the formal models.

Suburban also implemented evidence-based practices. Primary among them were supported employment services. However, a manager related to me that they did not adhere strictly to the formal model of the service:

> We're not spending as much time as the model suggests in helping a person identify what jobs they really want. The model says the people are going to stay in jobs longer if they've identified the job that they want to do. We tend to run with—if a client says, "I want to do this," we'll move heaven and earth to help him do that. Most clients, unfortunately, don't have a clue what they want to do, or have a very narrow-road view, and when presented with a job will say, "Yeah, that's the job for me!" And so a lot of clients get jobs that are available, not jobs that they've necessarily chosen. (interview)

Though that was the case, the organization was quite successful in obtaining community employment for clients they worked with. Another evidence-based practice the organization implemented during my research was illness management and recovery, a curriculum-based service that focused on clients setting and achieving concrete goals. One manager, Glenda, described the services as a "bunch of cognitive-behavioral stuff" (field notes). Workers described the formal evaluation of their use of the service during "fidelity visits" as "mixed," but staff who performed the service very much appreciated the clear guidelines they were given to follow, especially since the name of the service contained the vague buzzword "recovery." As one worker described it, those types of practices and evaluations gave them a much clearer sense of what to do than they received in many other areas of their work: "It's far more clear—less ambiguous. As stressful as those things can be, you get much clearer direction" (interview).

A final component of the logic of bureaucratic accountability that was perhaps felt most starkly by staff at the organization was a focus on *productivity*. As stated earlier, the shift in the funding mechanisms for public mental health services resulted in both organizations having to shift how they provided and tracked services. The autonomy and ability to be creative with services was severely restricted in the shift from grant funding to fee-for-service. Jade, a business manager at Urban, explained to me the message that became more and more important for her to relate to staff: "What I try to get across [is], basically, we're a not-for-profit business. But, you know what, we're a business. And we have to have our money coming in for us to provide our service and our business is providing services" (interview). So, in response to the impending changes in policy, the organization broke down productivity expectations for each individual worker, with possible sanctions for repeatedly missing them. Hours for the day program were even extended, primarily to increase the ability to bring in more clients for whom workers could bill (which reduced the amount of time staff had each day to complete documentation and other administrative work). The pressure was likewise felt at Suburban. The umbrella organization tracked billable hours closely and published reports regularly to let programs know how both the program and individual workers were doing in terms of billing expectations.

Workers at both organizations described the push for productivity as deeply affecting how they did their work. "You have to understand, Kerry, that now we're 'billing whores,'" one worker at Suburban related (field notes). Workers felt they had to gear their work toward what was billable. For example, Taylor, a worker at Urban, explained how he had to fight not to let billing requirements drive how he interacted with clients:

> I think the main—main tension I feel is . . . making sure that I'm not viewing the client as a productivity number. Um, I think it's always in the back of my mind, like I have to make this certain amount of . . . [billable] hours per month. And so . . . I just have to make sure . . . that I'm really executing quality clinical care on top of, you know, making sure I'm making my numbers. . . . I think I have to make that distinction in my mind a lot that . . . really dealing with folks for their clinical needs and how I can assist them . . . over [laughing] the dollar amount they are providing. (interview)

The different components of the logic were tightly interwoven. So the drive for documentation was in part motivated to justify continuing to bill for providing services to clients. Each act of documentation was a source of billing as well as a source of evaluation, both for "fidelity" evaluators and for auditors.

Type of Institutionalization

The central thrust of the logic of bureaucratic accountability is about *regulative* institutionalization. As was mentioned earlier, CARF served as a basis of both normative and regulative institutionalization for both Urban and Suburban— normative because of its field-level legitimizing role as an accrediting organization, and regulative because of its policy role in substituting for state oversight.

That is the case for empowerment as well. CARF's detailed standards manuals are updated and changed annually to deal with developments in mental health best practices. Furthermore, audits involved detailed investigations into a wide range of organizational practices, including documentation.

Regulative institutionalization was perhaps most evident, where I conducted my research, in changes in state mental health services policy. In addition to the previously mentioned changes to the state Medicaid mental health service definitions, the state also changed from a grant-based Medicaid funding system for community providers to a fee-for-service reimbursement system. There were a couple of notable effects of these changes for Urban and Suburban. First, more—and more detailed—documentation was required. Both organizations changed their computer systems to accommodate the change in policy. Before the change, PSR groups at Suburban required a staff member to complete one service note for all clients in the group. In addition, each PSR client received a monthly summary note on his or her progress in the program. After the change, however, these practices were replaced by a requirement for an individual note on each client in the group. Groups could have up to fifteen clients for each staff member and, given there were numerous groups in a day, the documentation increased dramatically. One worker at Suburban complained that it took her "forty-five minutes to do [the documentation on] a forty-five minute group" on the new system (field notes).

A second, related effect was an overall squeeze on organization finances—their funding levels would drop on the fee-for-service system if casework practices did not change to bring in more revenue. This led the organizations to increase the focus on productivity, developing internal policies to deal with these field-level changes, as noted above. The state's (and CARF's) audits enforced the regulations.

There were a couple of ways this logic was also normatively institutionalized at the field level. First, a wide range of organizations and stakeholders have endorsed reforming and monitoring the general and mental health care systems, despite disagreeing about which aspects need attention and how the activities should be carried out (Casalino 2004; Mechanic 2004; Scott et al. 2000). Two themes stand out: First, in both general health care and mental health care, the perceived need to close the gap between research and practice has taken the form of a normative imperative. For instance, the President's New Freedom Commission's final report devotes a section to explaining the following statements: "The Delay Is Too Long before Research Reaches Practice," "Too Few Benefit from Available Treatment," and "Reimbursement

Policies Do Not Foster Converting Research into Practice" (President's New Freedom Commission on Mental Health 2003). Further, the Evidence-Based Practices Project, begun in 2000, involved a major private-public partnership, including SAMHSA and the Robert Wood Johnson Foundation (as well as Dartmouth University). It also involved the executive director of the National Alliance for the Mentally Ill, a leading advocacy organization for people with mental illness and their families. The project worked on implementation strategies and tools for putting evidence-based practices into frontline mental health practice (Grob and Goldman 2007). The language evident in the IOM reports regarding the research-practice gap also points toward normative institutionalization: terms such as "failure" and "lack" are ubiquitous, demonstrating the viewpoint that the connection should be stronger and best practices should be driving care.

Second, cost containment has long been recognized as a problem in health care, though it has been addressed differently over the years (Scott et al. 2000). Governmental interest and efforts began when its role in funding greatly expanded after the passage of Medicaid and Medicare in the 1960s. Such interest has included the mental health care sector, as Medicaid has become a major funder for services for people with severe mental illness in the community (Day 2006; Mechanic 2007). Thus, whether it is individuals paying for mental health care out of their own pockets or the public paying for it out of their tax revenues, the need to rein in costs has been widely recognized, normatively institutionalized at the field level. Although various strategies to deal with costs might or might not be preferred by different segments of society, escalating costs have been seen as "a national problem" since at least the 1960s (Mechanic 2004). Urban and Suburban had to comply with the logic (and force their workers to do so) in order to be considered a legitimate provider, but normative institutionalization was not evident inside the organizations.

Conclusion

These logics were experienced by workers as constraints—conscious or unconscious—on their thoughts, actions, or behaviors. Several agents of institutionalization played major roles in most or all of the logics, such as state policy and CARF. Moreover, CARF helped to institutionalize the logics through both normative and regulative means because of its legitimizing function and its distinct relationship with state policy.

At times the logics reinforced each other, such as with regulative elements like the Supreme Court's *Olmstead* decision, which was steeped in both the community and empowerment logics, allowing clients to have a voice in deciding when they were ready for more independence. During these times, workers could take solace in the definitiveness of courses of action, whether they personally agreed with them or not. However, at other times, logics pulled workers toward conflicting courses of action, and the best way forward was not all that obvious. For instance, what happens when a client chooses dependence? The empowerment logic dictated respecting client choice; however, the community logic argued against that choice if workers thought the client was "ready." The following chapters will deal with these types of institutional fragmentation and will consider how the nature of the logics themselves, along with creative, "street-level" adaptive practices, determines outcomes in those situations.

Chapter 3

Diagnosis, Labeling, and Social Control

Though you would never know it by interacting with him, Frankie Young has been involved with the mental health system on and off for decades. In fact, he met his now-deceased wife of twenty-five years through this involvement—they met when they were both residents in a "halfway house" for people with mental illness. His wife's death threw his life into upheaval, both emotionally and financially. "I wanted to kill myself. . . . I had a gun to my head," he said. He lost his home and lived on the street for several years. Outreach workers for Urban encountered him on the street, and he became involved in their programming.

But a deeper look into Frankie's mental health history—and the way Urban's workers talked about him—revealed ambiguity about what exactly his mental problems were, and how much any problems he did have actually impaired his ability to live a productive life. He had been given several different primary diagnoses. During my research, he was consistently diagnosed with major depression in psychiatric evaluations, but workers were unclear about the nature and severity of Frankie's problems. One of his workers said they were "throwing around" his diagnosis. When he first became involved with Urban, several years before my research there began, his depression diagnosis was combined with a diagnosis of alcohol dependence and personality disorder not otherwise specified (NOS). These official diagnoses remained for most of his time with Urban. He was prescribed antidepressants, and he said he took them regularly. Psychiatric reports showed his condition was good; one psychiatrist wrote that Frankie "is not symptomatic." However, the combination of staff concerns regarding some of his far-fetched, uncorroborated claims and a change of psychiatrists at Urban led to a change in his official diagnosis near the end of my time there. The depression diagnosis remained, but his other diagnoses became psychosis NOS and a "rule out" diagnosis of delusional disorder.[1] This was coupled with a new prescription for antipsychotic medication, which he had not been prescribed for decades.

In day-to-day organizational life, this ambiguity regarding Frankie's diagnosis caused little concern for workers at Urban. His history of psychiatric hospitalization and previous use of antipsychotic medication made it easy to justify, bureaucratically, his being there. Plus, they had very few problems with him. When his name came up in worker meetings, though conversations might involve workers' amused reflections on his wild claims, he was rarely brought up in discussions regarding disruption or violence. Actually, workers saw him as quite dependable and frequently enlisted his help in completing necessary tasks around the day program, such as preparing lunch. On top of his helping out at Urban, Frankie also worked as a janitor at a local nursing facility, where he was paid "off the books." His schedule was unpredictable and flexible, but he often spoke of working on a regular basis. Nevertheless, the income from this job was not sufficient to live on, and he had no medical coverage. He had a painful ulcer that required surgery, but he had no means to pay for it. Urban and local public aid lawyers were helping him reapply for Social Security work disability benefits and Medicaid, both of which he had been denied in the past. It was common for clients of Urban to be denied benefits and to reapply numerous times, with help and encouragement from Urban.

From Frankie's perspective, there was no doubt he was depressed since his wife died. Beyond that, he did not regularly describe other symptoms of mental illness. Regardless of symptoms he experienced—or didn't—his involvement in the mental health system had shown him that having a mental illness diagnosis could qualify him for resources otherwise unavailable. For instance, at one time both Frankie and his wife apparently called on these resources by seeking shelter in a mental hospital. A discharge report from this hospitalization states, "Patient is exuberant and shows no signs of depression or other mental illness. . . . Patient admitted that he and his wife cooked up the stories about being suicidal because they had no other place to go."

One day as I exited Urban's building, I saw Frankie down the street speaking to someone I didn't know. I walked down to say hi. I greeted him and met his friend. As usual, Frankie was wearing well-worn clothes and a ball cap with wisps of long and rapidly thinning hair shooting out from under it. In his

trademark fashion, he talked quickly. After each point he made, he immediately turned around and took a few steps away, only to turn right back around
and continue talking. He tended to repeat this process over and over during
conversations. You would know he was done talking to you when he didn't
turn back around. Maybe he would say good-bye; maybe he wouldn't.

This day, I asked how his application for Social Security benefits was
going. He showed me a letter that stated he had to meet with a government-
designated psychiatrist to determine his eligibility. A worker from Urban was
going to go to the appointment with him. The psychiatrist would conduct an
evaluation and might assign Frankie a diagnosis. The results of the evaluation
would play a major role in Social Security's decision of whether to approve
Frankie's application for benefits. In the past he had attempted to qualify based
solely on physical disabilities but had been unsuccessful.

Frankie realized how important the psychiatric evaluation was, and what
kind of results would lead to an increased likelihood of receiving benefits. "I've
got to tell them . . . you know, I got leprechauns in my house. I keep them in
my closet," he said with a half smile, wide-eyed. He turned away, took a few
steps, and then came back. He said he had to prove to them that "I don't have
all my marbles." I asked about his diagnosis; was it depression? He said he was
diagnosed as "a leprechaun specialist," again with the wry smile. On a later day
when I asked him about the visit with the psychiatrist, Frankie said he liked the
doctor. "He was a down-to-earth guy," he said. "[The doctor] thinks I should
get something. . . . He said he doesn't know what [Social Security is] gonna do.
. . . All they wanted him to do is his diagnosis." I asked Frankie what the diagnosis ended up being. He said, somewhat hesitantly, "I, ah, I'm a little—that I
am little depressed and everything. He said I could, probably, say I hallucinate
things, that my wife is there. I think he had to put something there." It seems
that, like Frankie, the psychiatrist understands the importance of a diagnosis of
severe mental illness.

Assigning an "accurate" official diagnosis in community mental health services
is no simple matter. Though a casual perusal of the American Psychiatric Association's *Diagnostic and Statistical Manual of Mental Disorders* (*DSM*) may
make it seem a cookie-cutter process, in actual practice that can be far from the
case. Clinical "best practice" manuals emphasize the importance of "getting to
know" patients, understanding and contextualizing their experience to see if
they actually merit clinical significance. As Frankie's story shows, with new

information, diagnoses can change. The clinical-professional logic dictates that not just anyone can or should carry out this task, either. Only a mental health care worker with expert clinical certification should (or could, by state law) officially assign a diagnosis.

At Urban and Suburban, applying an official label of mental illness was a formal, discrete organizational event. Though such labels were reviewed at regular intervals, each review likewise was a discrete, bureaucratic event. These labels were initially applied through the client intake process. Various organization staff met with clients, obtaining any available documentation from previous providers. Paperwork was then completed, detailing the clients' social and mental health histories as well as their current needs, desires, and functioning. The resulting label regarding diagnosis and severity of illness became the official line in all organizational documentation.

Quite aside from examining the assignment of these official diagnoses, one may ask what purpose they serve once applied. As examples of the application of expert clinical knowledge, ideally they function as the signposts guiding clinical interventions (Jutel 2009). More broadly, studies such as that by Erving Goffman argue that these official diagnoses mediated nearly all interactions between patients and staff in the mental hospital "total institutions" that used to dominate mental health treatment (Goffman 1961). In a process Goffman refers to as "looping," for instance, patients' protests to their treatment in the hospital were themselves reacted to as symptoms of their mental illness. So, a patient's claims of repeated mistreatment by workers might be seen as paranoia, or "the bitter comments he made in a letter to a sibling—a letter which the recipient has forwarded to the hospital administrator, [might] be added to the patient's dossier and brought along to the conference" (37) (see also Rosenhan 1973).

However, as Frankie's story also reveals, official labels serve many functions beyond guiding clinical judgments and interactions. As Annemarie Jutel and Sarah Nettleton (2011:793) explain, diagnosis also "provides access to key resources and facilitates their allocation." So those to whom the resources would be distributed—often clients like Frankie and mental health care organizations like Urban—as well as those distributing, are very interested in diagnoses. Third-party payers often require diagnosis for payment (P. Brown 1987; Kirk and Kutchins 1988; Kirk and Kutchins 1992; Wilson 1993), at times pegging the amount of payment to the given diagnosis, as in diagnosis-related groups. Having a severe mental illness diagnosis acknowledged by the state would allow Frankie to be designated as having a disability and would qualify him for Social Security benefits and medical coverage for his ulcer.

Official diagnosis is not the only way mental health workers classify clients. They also informally classify clients, and these informal labels are as important as the official diagnostic ones in determining what occurs in day-to-day life in mental health care. For instance, Frankie was not defined solely through his diagnosis; he was also seen by workers as dependable and helpful. Ivan Belknap (1956) observed that such informal classifications of patients based on "their manageability and occupational utility" were more significant than psychiatric diagnosis in the daily management of the mental hospital (128). A variety of pragmatic classifications can outweigh staff's clinical classifications in determining workers' treatments of clients (Emerson and Pollner 1978; Floersch 2000; Peyrot 1982).

At Urban and Suburban, although official diagnoses were ideally an application of the clinical-professional logic, in practice they were appropriated to serve the demands of the logic of bureaucratic accountability. Workers adapted to this situation by using the clinical-professional logic to apply informal labels of mental illness, which they saw as more accurate, to clients. These combined with informal labels regarding client disruption to allow workers to both meet funding demands and manage everyday organizational life.

Official Mental Illness Labels: Necessity and Limitations

The clinical-professional logic dictates that clinicians can and should use their expert knowledge to make sense of clients' experiences clinically, but there are issues that make it practically impossible for this type of understanding to occur prior to diagnosis. Informational shortfalls, combined with incentives to quickly assign severe official labels of mental illness, led clinicians to assign diagnoses that were expedient and, at times, transparently incorrect. First, obtaining clients' mental health histories was a difficult, long-term process. One issue was that clients often did not feel comfortable discussing important information with strangers. This was especially the case if clients had been homeless, had had no previous contact with the mental health system, or had been out of the mental health system for a long period of time; these factors were encountered more often at Urban. Jonas, an outreach worker for Urban, described how clients' lack of trust could prevent workers from gaining information they needed to make accurate diagnoses: "It's a very difficult task. . . . Homeless people, because of their fears, or maybe sometimes because of their paranoia, they move from [place to place] and they're hard to follow up with. . . . Often because of the stigma in society, people still have shame, of course. They would be hesitant to say they were in [psychiatric hospitals], so there's a challenge to be observant [for symptoms]" (interview). Aware of the possibility for stigmatization from labeling, potential clients could be guarded in interaction. Shauntee, a client at Urban, described feeling this way in her first encounter with Urban's outreach workers: "I was at the Salvation Army. . . . They said to me, 'Hi, how are you doing? We have a new program that's openin' up.' And they asked me, do I think I have any mental issues. At first I was like, leery, because I didn't really know them" (interview). Initial distrust could be hard to overcome, and true openness from clients might not occur until well after they began receiving services from the organization.

Even if clients were willing to discuss their lives and problems openly with workers, information could still be limited. This is because of a second issue: documents giving important details about clients' previous contacts with the mental health system were often difficult to locate or obtain. For potential clients who were homeless or whose mental health history was unclear, the initial interview by outreach or intake workers was essential. Unfortunately, this was sometimes the only source of information about the client for a while. In such cases, workers were encouraged to "just go on their [clients'] word" regarding their history, as one worker from Suburban said. For clients referred to the organizations from other service providers, as was more common at Suburban, the situation could be somewhat better, as the other organization was sure to have a file, however limited, on the prospective client. Even that documentation might only record the client's stay in that organization, and lack prior history. Generally, though, the previous organization had done at least some search for other paperwork, which Urban or Suburban could then supplement with their own searches. In spite of these efforts, client files were nearly always incomplete (given clients' own stated mental health history) and were at times very sparse.

Granted, the value of a relatively complete client file was questionable, given the changes in diagnostic practices and fashions over time and the variation between organizations and between different clinicians in diagnosis. As the range of diagnoses and treatments given to Frankie shows, a complete file could be more befuddling than enlightening (cf. Bittner and Garfinkle 1967). Nevertheless, workers preferred more information to less, and they were rarely satisfied with what they received.

A third issue that made applying an accurate diagnosis difficult was that clients might have different reasons for requesting services than organizations had in providing them. For organizations, the official linchpin of all other services was client mental illness. Clients, however, might not see themselves as mentally ill, or might not see their mental illness as their primary problem.

Having a safe place to spend time, socialize, obtain low-cost or free food, or have "something to do" other than "sit at home" were all incentives that drew clients to the organizations. More broadly, many clients saw social services as their reason for becoming involved, frequently citing housing and vocational services as major concerns. Clients often viewed such benefits as ends in themselves, whereas organizations frequently framed them as means of "engaging" clients in order to obtain their consent for mental health treatment.

For example, consider the case of Karl, a prospective client at Suburban whose intake meeting I attended. Karl lived in a residential mental health services organization, but was considering obtaining some services from Suburban as well. He talked with worker Monique, who asked him why he wanted to join. Karl said he wanted housing. Monique asked if that was the only reason. He replied no, he wanted to grow, to find out more about himself (field notes). But a little over a week later, I was in the office with Harvey, the worker who ended up assigned to Karl. He was talking to Karl; Karl had decided he did not want to join the program. After he hung up the phone, Harvey told me that Karl had "some interesting reasons" for not wanting to join the program. He said he really only wanted independent housing, not groups and the other components of the program. Harvey said, "He said he can pursue those housing goals there at [his residential] program and have more time for himself" (field notes). Though Karl was receiving mental health services elsewhere, this example shows that clients and the organization might not see eye to eye on what the clients stand to gain from joining a program. The important point here is that clients' lack of agreement with staff about their needs could impede clinicians assigning an informed official label.

The extreme example of this mismatch of official organizational goals and client desires occurred when the client feigned or exaggerated symptoms in order to receive social services. Given the often more desperate situation of potential clients at Urban, this practice was only reported to me at this site. At Suburban, some clients had personal connections to people in the organizational hierarchy, connections they could use to obtain job services from the organization without being mentally ill; feigning mental illness was not necessary for them. At Urban, though, such connections usually were absent. Instead, potential clients used their connections to other clients to learn what was necessary to receive certain services. Like Frankie, these clients learned the importance of a diagnosis of severe mental illness. Bobby, a worker at Urban, observed, "You'd be surprised in a community how the word [regarding resources and how to obtain them] gets around right away" (interview).

In addition to these issues in obtaining truthful and complete information necessary to understand a client's mental health, workers also faced two incentives to apply a diagnosis to potential clients as quickly as possible. First, official diagnoses played a major role in complying with the documentation and productivity components of the logic of bureaucratic accountability, thus affecting resource flows for the organizations. As mentioned, mental health care organizations had to comply with a large (and increasing) number of rules and procedures to ensure continued funding from the state, and the official diagnosis was a key component of many of these.

An example of the importance of official diagnoses for bureaucratic accountability was their major role in proving the "medical necessity" of serving clients, a condition of government reimbursement. As a documentation "best practices" manual from Suburban explained, "'medical necessity' is derived from the medical model," which is based on "defining the problems a person is experiencing in the form of symptoms, behaviors and impairments." Only when such transformation from problems to "sickness" had taken place would Medicaid—a *medical* insurance program—pay for services addressing clients' problems. This necessity for diagnosis led one worker at Urban to refer to the APA's *Diagnostic and Statistical Manual of Mental Disorders* as "our little book of witchcraft so we can bill" (field notes).

Community mental health care organizations like Urban and Suburban that serve the chronically mentally ill provide many social services such as housing, vocational services, and help in obtaining public assistance, in addition to providing psychiatric services (Cook and Wright 1995; Cuddeback and Morrissey 2010; Estroff 1981; Floersch 2000; Goldman and Morrissey 1985). With the rollback of services in other sectors of the public welfare system in the United States, mental health services broadly—and mental illness disability designation in particular—have become ways to provide help that might be otherwise difficult to provide to those in need (Watkins-Hayes 2009; cf. Peyrot 1991). Although this is the case, the logic of bureaucratic accountability constrains organizations such as Urban and Suburban in how—and to whom—they provide these services.

Applying official diagnoses of severe mental illness met these demands. Although organizations might find supplemental sources of funding that allowed them to serve small numbers of clients who they did not label severely mentally ill, these tended to be exceptions. Though patchworks of grant funding could help plug holes and drive innovation, Medicaid was the major source of stable funding for the organizations. Demonstrating these constraints, a manager at

Suburban described how his hands were largely tied in how he provided services. He said one of the major issues was that "we've made everything medical," when a great deal of what they provided were social services. He said the state would not pay for social services, though (field notes). It would not pay for social services, that is, unless those services were made *medical* services.

So in order to be reimbursed by Medicaid for providing services, Urban and Suburban had to officially label incoming clients *severely mentally ill*. State Medicaid policy divided the client population into two groups: eligible and target. To become "eligible" to receive services, clients had to be given a diagnosis from a ten-page list of Axis I or Axis II diagnoses from the *Diagnostic and Statistical Manual of Mental Disorders*, fourth edition.[2] These clients were not viewed as a top priority in policy and so the state said they "may be served, contingent on availability of resources." Mental retardation, non-dual-diagnosed substance abuse disorders, and some "organic disorders" such as dementia were excluded from the list. In addition to assigning a diagnosis, in order to qualify the client as eligible, the organization had to demonstrate that the client's illness caused significant impairment in functioning. The criteria for the "target" population—which were the groups seen as top priority for treatment—were even more stringent, allowing only thirteen types of disorders.[3] It also required demonstrating both an intensive mental health treatment history and more severe functional impairment. Not all organizations in the state were funded to serve both populations. The state funded Suburban to serve both target and eligible populations, whereas Urban was funded to serve only the target population.[4] In either case, however, qualifying for services meant the organization officially labeled the client as severely mentally ill.

Although the clinical-professional logic dictated applying clinical expertise to "accurately" diagnose clients, the information problems and countervailing pressures of bureaucratic accountability could lead the clinician to assign a diagnosis even when no clear signs of a given illness were present. This issue was raised by a psychiatric provider at Suburban in her discussion of initial mental health screenings:

> As far as a diagnosis, I mean you could come up with a diagnosis for anyone, I suppose—you know, Depression NOS, or Adjustment Disorder . . . and that's kind of the difficult thing at some places, too, because, yeah, you see someone for an evaluation. . . . And, you know, you feel, well, they have some depressive symptoms but they function okay and they don't need, they don't want treatment at this point. Well, for billing

purposes every office requires you put down something, you know. So, you can't bill Medicare [or Medicaid] with no diagnosis. So then you have to put down something. So a lot of times just maybe [you'll put down], you know, Depression NOS 'cause they have couple depressive symptoms. You know, certainly you don't hope that a diagnosis like that sticks with them. (interview)

Though the provider noted reluctance to apply the label based on clinical criteria and the stigmatizing effects of mental illness labels, she also describes the organizational incentive—or unspoken imperative— to label clients mentally ill. At Urban this process was affected by the organization's significant homeless outreach services. These services were involved in trying to engage potential clients, to make later official engagement (and labeling) possible. Thus, it was not uncommon for services to be provided to clients without them (yet) having a severely mentally ill label, at least for short periods of time. The pressure to officially label was nevertheless noticeable in relieved or triumphant expressions I observed accompanying workers' reports of finally officially labeling clients and registering them for services. For instance, at one intake meeting at Urban, it was announced that a client who was receiving services but had not yet been officially labeled finally had a completed mental health assessment. Jessica, a manager in the day program, quickly asked if she could have a copy. Another worker observed of Jessica, "She'll hunt you down" for paperwork, which brought a great deal of laughter. Jessica explained her persistence: she needed to bill for the services she provided and could not do so until she had all the paperwork—including the mental health assessment formally assigning a diagnosis—to register the client (field notes).

A second incentive to apply official labels of severe mental illness to clients was that many who worked for these organizations—especially Urban— were motivated to serve a broader population than their resource streams would permit (cf. Peyrot 1991). They wanted to help the disadvantaged—not just that subsection with severe mental illness. Although only those labeled severely mentally ill qualified for assistance, the services available—especially the social services—would be helpful also to those not so labeled. Urban had a small grant from the state Division of Alcohol and Substance Abuse, but as one manager stated, "Even that's for people that are dually diagnosed [with mental illness and substance use disorder]" (interview). Facing such barriers to service provision, clinicians could act on their commitment to serve clients by officially labeling them. One psychiatric provider at Urban described a strategy of manipulating diagnoses: "Because of the population we serve, we have a public—public agenda. And I think that a lot of us would rather see somebody housed with support and will make the diagnosis fit. . . . I have done it and I—I look at some of these charts and I know that some of the docs before me had done it." (interview).

These incentives to serve those in need could at times have a less idealistic and a more practical bent to them. At Suburban, some of the most in-demand resources provided to clients were the vocational services, which had a remarkable track record of success in connecting clients with jobs. So successful was the organization that many wanted to make use of the services for prospective clients who were not inarguably mentally ill. For instance, the state Department of Rehabilitation Services (DORS) often referred clients with mental illness to Suburban for vocational services, which it paid Suburban for providing. The success Suburban had in working with these clients motivated DORS to work out a special contract with Suburban to work with "difficult" clients who did not have severe mental illness. However, because they did not have an official severe mental illness label, the clients were not fully integrated into the organization's services. The mental health workers there could not be reimbursed for working with those clients, thus depriving vocational workers of additional support in handling client problems. When clients became increasingly difficult to work with, there was a motivation for vocational workers to have an official severe mental illness label applied to the clients so they could gain extra support from the mental health workers. Jane, a vocational worker at Suburban, described finding justification to label a DORS-referred client with a physical disability as severely mentally ill. "DORS referred me a non-MI [not mentally ill] client and [he] ended up being an MI client because he had so many problems. . . . We further investigated, like, his paperwork at the nursing home, and found about nine diagnoses that this guy had, most of which were physical—all the way from lower back pain to leg areas. . . . There was tucked in there a bipolar disorder [diagnosis]" (interview). Jane used that diagnosis to satisfy the logic of bureaucratic accountability's demands for a label to open the client for mental health services and gained extra support in managing the case.

It's clear that official labels of severe mental illness, although often the hinge on which all mental health care hangs, in actuality are sometimes more a bureaucratic tool than an actual clinical depiction of a client's condition. This fact limits the labels' usefulness in managing interactions with clients on a day-to-day basis. Instead, informal labels of both client mental illness and of how disruptive clients are to organizational rules and routines allow workers to implement the clinical logic and manage everyday organizational life.

Informal Labels: The Management of Organizational Life

Carol Heimer and Lisa Staffen (1995, 1998) describe how workers in neo-natal intensive care units label parents of children on the unit based on the "clinical" issue of their ability to provide adequate care for their child's medical condition but also on more practical issues regarding how disruptive they are to the units' routines. I found that workers at Urban and Suburban similarly applied two different types of informal labels to clients: informal clinical labels of mental illness and informal labels of client disruption. Agreement on these informal labels might not be shared by every single staff member, but they were generally shared by most. Significantly, informal clinical labels could conflict with official clinical labels in their construction of client mental illness.

As with official labels of mental illness, staff also informally labeled clients as either *severely mentally ill* or *not severely mentally ill.* These informal labels were similar to official ones in that they took into account both symptoms expressed (which might or might not in informal cases be discussed in terms of diagnosis) and the amount of functional impairment caused by the symptoms. However, informal labels differed from official ones in important ways. First, informal labels were continually negotiated among staff, having no formal benchmarks for review. Realizing the limited utility of official diagnoses, staff members, in meetings, case conferences, and day-to-day conversations about clients, discussed clients' diagnosis and functioning as independent of their official assigned labels.

A second difference between official and informal labels of mental illness was that although informal labels greatly impacted client treatment, changes in them did not necessarily threaten formal resource flows. Whereas changing a client's official label of mental illness might disqualify them from Medicaid-reimbursable services, changing their informal labels to not severely mentally ill (and leaving the official label as severely mentally ill) allowed staff to change their behavior toward clients while still providing some services and billing the state for them. Informal labels of mental illness served different purposes than official labels: official labels situated the client in the organizational bureaucracy (meeting the demands of bureaucratic accountability) and opened up resource flows; informal labels dictated how staff reacted to and interacted with clients on a day-to-day basis, allowing them to implement the clinical-professional logic more freely.

Highlighting the fragmented nature of labeling, workers' official and informal labels of severe mental illness for the same client could clash. The very workers who regularly applied (or reproduced) official labels of severe client mental illness in organizational documentation might in a casual conversation with other staff discuss how the client did not appear to be severely mentally ill. Aside from such cases of transparent official mislabeling as discussed earlier, staff's impression of clients sometimes changed over time. For example, a staff member might note a reduction in the symptoms of illness clients expressed, though the client was not taking medication. In this way, the informal label might not necessarily be viewed as reflecting an immutable aspect of the client. Rather, the label was the construction of client functioning under specific circumstances. Because many of the incentives for officially labeling the client severely mentally ill in the first place persisted once the client became part of the organization (that is, the need for billable services and the mission to serve those in need), staff could not simply change the label to align with evolving impressions of the client.[5]

In addition to informally labeling client mental illness, staff also informally labeled clients based on how well they adhered to rules and routines and how much disruption they caused. Day-to-day life in Urban and Suburban involved rules and expectations of clients. Staff expected clients to show up at the organization or to their appointments. Clients were to attempt to get along with each other and with staff and to resolve disagreements relatively peacefully. Above all, however, clients were to respect staff expertise and discretion by following staff direction and redirection. At Urban, these expectations were most visible during incidents involving safety, such as threats or actual violent confrontations, which occurred on average a couple of times a month. At Suburban, in contrast, violence was extremely rare (only two incidents occurred during my seven months of fieldwork). Informal labels of disruption at Suburban were more commonly tied to the mundane, day-to-day activities that required less effort from staff and were more rewarding (financially, practically, or therapeutically) if clients complied. Examples included group attendance, not talking while staff or other clients were talking, and keeping scheduled appointments (at Urban these issues, though sometimes buried by the more stark episodes mentioned, could inform labels as well).

If clients were compliant with these rules and routines, staff informally labeled them *directable* or *not problem clients* or *not disruptive.* If they were not, staff would label them *problem clients* or *disruptive or not directable.* These labels were assigned independent of any official or unofficial labels of mental illness. Regardless of the cause to which staff attributed the disruption—illness

Table 3.1. Informal Labeling and Social Control of Clients in Community
Mental Health Services

General staff label	Informal label of mental illness	Informal label of client disruption	Type of social control
Good	Not severely mentally ill Severely mentally ill	Not disruptive	NA
Bad	Not severely mentally ill	Disruptive	Exclusionary
Symptomatic	Severely mentally ill	Disruptive	Integrative

or willful deviance, for example—it was the perceived pattern of disruption that elicited the label from staff.

There were three overarching labels staff applied to clients (refer to table 3.1). Some clients rarely or infrequently caused disruptions and were seen as *good* clients. When clients repeatedly violated organizational rules and routines, informal organizational labels of mental illness determined how staff dealt with them. Workers acted differently toward disruptive clients based on whether they were informally labeled *severely mentally ill* or *not severely mentally ill*: depending on the label, a client was either *symptomatic* or *bad*, which determined the type of social control applied.[6]

The Good

Clients who were informally labeled as not disruptive were seen as so-called good clients. Because they were not disruptive to the organization, they were not subject to much social control. In fact, these clients could be quite helpful to have around the organization. They were sometimes enlisted as dependable free labor, carrying out routine tasks around the organizations such as making lunch, as Frankie often did. However, the single label, good, could have a couple of distinct meanings, depending on workers' informal labels regarding client mental illness.

When clients were informally labeled as not severely mentally ill, a moral valence was added to staff evaluations. Much as Talcott Parsons (1951) based his explanation of the sick role on the assumption that patients were involuntarily sick and wanted to get better, workers at Urban and Suburban thought these clients were better able to control their behaviors than clients truly thought to be severely mentally ill, and they expected them to use that ability. When they were seen as not disruptive, workers judged them to be morally fit and would be willing to serve them; being labeled good, for these clients, reflected staff's positive moral judgment of them. Frankie received this type of label from the staff at Urban. For most of my time there, Frankie's diagnosis was ambiguous to staff but was not a subject of much concern, informally speaking. Although near the end of my research staff became concerned about his possibly delusional statements, they never thought him severely impaired. Moreover, because he was helpful and not disruptive, workers were willing to serve him in the organization and even assist him in seeking additional benefits through Social Security and Medicaid.

The good label could also be applied to clients who were labeled as severely mentally ill and as not disruptive. These clients were exempt from moral evaluation. Here the label of good denoted not a moral label but simply a statement that clients were not generally problem-causing and generally did what workers thought they were supposed to do. Workers saw these clients— for example, those who sat quietly and muttered or laughed to themselves instead of yelling or threatening others—as still suffering from serious symptoms of mental illness, but not the kind that would lead to many disruptions of organizational rules or routines. Barney, a client who lived at Suburban's residence and occasionally attended the day program, was labeled in this way. Barney was diagnosed with schizoaffective disorder and obsessive-compulsive disorder. His condition had improved markedly over the years he had spent at Suburban. As one worker, Monique, described, "This guy was catatonic. . . . He. Did. Not. Speak" (field notes). Over time, he came to speak, and he had held a job as grocery store packer for several years when I met him. However, workers thought he still had some serious mental health issues. Specifically, he had problems coping with his anxiety symptoms. He had a tendency to avoid social interaction and isolate himself. Despite these issues, Barney was very compliant with staff direction, doing basically whatever workers asked him to do. He was known as one of the dependable clients at the group home, one who could be counted on when other clients could not, though he sometimes needed worker assistance. Furthermore, even though he tended to socially isolate, Barney went on activities with other members of the group home. Because of this compliance despite his symptoms, Barney was labeled a good client. Like Frankie, Barney was not subject to major social control efforts.

The Bad

At times, clients who were informally labeled as not severely mentally ill were also labeled as disruptive; staff believed these clients could do better than they were doing. Because, unlike Frankie and some other so-called good clients, these clients were not exercising their imputed ability, staff saw them as morally culpable for not doing so. These were *bad* clients. Thus, workers permitted clients labeled in this way to violate rules and routines less frequently and to a lesser degree than those labeled as severely mentally ill. Staff dealt with these clients by reasoning with them—at times in a therapeutic manner, but if that was not successful, with ultimatums. Workers brought up issues of medication less frequently with these clients. If these clients took medication at all, they rarely took antipsychotics, which were the most effective drugs for handling disruptive behavior. More important, however, was that medication was not brought up because staff saw their issues as matters of will and of morality, neither of which medication could address.

So-called bad clients were subject to *exclusionary social control*. This type of social control was motivated by the belief that, if the client would not eliminate the behavior (which, again, workers saw as possible), then workers needed to eliminate the client. Though the client might be referred to other more or less intensive services from another organization, an exit could occur without such referrals. Client exits through this type of control were at times made without arranging services from another provider. Further, client exits could initially be short term (being "on restriction"), or they could be long term, especially if there had been previous exits due to problem behaviors. Exclusion here was seen as both a punishment and an opportunity for the client to make the choice to pay more attention to the rules and routines of the organization.

At other times, clients informally labeled as not severely mentally ill were viewed by workers as having an actual mental illness, but not a "severe" one that tremendously impacted their ability to function in the world. Some of their disruptions could be framed by workers as symptoms of mental disorder, but they would not be absolved of moral judgment by this fact. This type of informal labeling frequently involved clients viewed as having a personality disorder. Symptoms of personality disorders are seen as more long term, deeply ingrained, and diffused across more components of a person's life than the typical clinical disorders in Axis I of the *DSM IV*. Thus, clients who were frequently involved in disruptions but who were not viewed as exhibiting symptoms of Axis I disorders such as psychotic disorders or mood disorders were occasionally discussed as suffering from a personality disorder (which is on Axis II of the *DSM IV*). Borderline personality disorder was the most frequently discussed disorder in these circumstances.

At Urban, many staff seriously doubted the official label of Rodney. Though Rodney's official psychiatric diagnoses were paranoid schizophrenia and schizoaffective disorder (on different evaluations), workers did not discuss his behaviors in terms of being symptoms of these disorders, other than to argue that he was misdiagnosed. Rodney himself claimed he "stretched" (that is, exaggerated) his symptoms to get services from Urban, and he refused to take medication (interview). Workers frequently discussed his actions as symptoms of personality disorder. For example, Rodney consistently had conflicts (and eventually a physical altercation) with another client. During a meeting, one worker, Travis, said that the other client had decided to avoid Rodney in order to try to prevent further problems. The worker pointed out, "Rodney did not decide that, which brings up the Axis II issues again" (field notes). Recall that, as discussed above, being diagnosed with a personality disorder would not qualify Rodney for Medicaid-reimbursable services from Urban.

Though workers thought Rodney might have a mental illness, they still viewed him as able to control his behaviors. Several times I witnessed workers both threaten to and actually carry through with kicking him out of both individual groups and Urban's day program for a time. Rodney complained that he was held to a different standard than other clients were held to. He said that when he did the same thing other clients did, he was singled out. As an example, he pointed to a group that a worker named Pete was running and noted how all kinds of people were talking in it. Rodney said when he talked Pete "almost kicked me out" (field notes). Many workers freely admitted that they singled Rodney out. At one staff meeting, Jessica said she told Rodney that she understood his point regarding differential treatment, but that staff really tried to "see where people are at, and what they're capable of." Another worker, Steve, replied—to those present in the meeting, but as if speaking to Rodney— "That and, are you psychotic? I don't think so. Does anybody believe your Axis I diagnosis—paranoid schizophrenia? I don't think so" (field notes). Because his disruptions were considered a matter of will, not ability, Rodney was held to a higher standard and was subject to exclusionary social control.

Other clients labeled as not severely mentally ill were judged not to have any symptoms of mental illness. Jabar, a client at Suburban, was an example of this type of client. Though Jabar was officially diagnosed with schizoaffective disorder and was on several types of psychotropic medications, psychiatric evaluations described him as reporting that he experienced no symptoms of mental illness (though they described him as delusional regarding his past). During my fieldwork at Suburban, I never observed workers describe Jabar's problematic behavior as symptoms of mental illness. Instead, it was framed as behavior that he was willingly participating in and could control. For example, Suzanne, a worker at the house where Jabar lived, talked about "just [feeling] so sorry" that she could not reason with another resident of the house. This other resident with a psychotic disorder was disruptive, unmedicated, highly symptomatic, and refused to participate in most services Suburban offered. However, when Suzanne talked about Jabar and his refusals and disruptions, her tone was quite different: "Everybody else is maintaining their recovery, and they're basically not here. And mostly [the only time] you can . . . find the clients all at home at the same time is after six o'clock, and that's the end of their day, whether they are working in school or coming from the [day program].That person that I spoke about that's refusing the program [Jabar], he just lays around, eats, sleeps, and smokes cigarettes. I'm trying to get him back in program" (interview).

Staff labeled Jabar as a bad client. In meetings, staff argued that they needed to hold Jabar accountable. Workers judged Jabar as able to control his disruptive behaviors. Jabar pointed to the different standard to which his unmedicated, disruptive housemate was held. Although Suburban rarely involuntarily terminated services with clients due to organizational policy, they were at times less assertive in maintaining services for disruptive clients, or even encourage those clients to leave services voluntarily. Thus, Jabar sensed that the encouragement he had received from workers to move out into his own apartment might have been motivated less by their thinking that it was in his best interest and more by how much easier it would make their jobs. Jabar talked about his interactions with a particular worker: "This is a big thing for him now. He'll wait a month, two, three months and ask me when I'm moving out [again]. I say, 'Well, have you asked [the unmedicated housemate] when she's moving out?' [The worker says,] 'We're not discussing [her]. When I get to [her] and if we discuss it, I'll tell her who is asking.' I said, 'Well man, you can be so childish to be so old.' . . . Because it was childish. . . . I'm too old for this shit" (interview). In meetings, workers at Suburban constantly discussed ways to overcome Jabar's resistance to organizational rules and routines and were, to some degree, at a loss. This, when considered with my observations of responses to other disruptive clients, makes Jabar's statement plausible, even though I did not observe multiple workers directly state a strategy of solving their problems by pushing Jabar to move out.

The Symptomatic

Staff informally labeled most clients as severely mentally ill. When these clients repeatedly violated rules and routines, and hence were labeled as disruptive, staff medicalized the actions, seeing them as the involuntary symptoms of a clinical disorder (Conrad and Schneider 1992). Unlike with so-called bad clients—including those perceived to have a mental illness—workers did not view these clients as willfully engaging in the behaviors, and they were absolved from moral evaluation. They were simply *symptomatic.*

Symptomatic clients were given more leeway in the violation of rules and routines before social control machinery kicked in. For the same violations, staff gave these clients either no sanctions or much less severe ones than those of other clients. For instance, I witnessed very different responses to clients assaulting one another, depending on whether those involved were labeled as bad or as symptomatic. In either case the altercation needed to be defused, of course. After that occurred, however, paths diverged. Symptomatic clients might receive no long-term consequences, whereas bad clients could be barred from the day program for a time.

For symptomatic clients, workers applied *integrative social control* (Braithwaite 1989; Heimer and Staffen 1995). Though workers were definitely motivated to contain disruptive and dangerous behaviors, they saw those behaviors as symptoms, which needed to be treated. This treatment was what the organization aimed for; thus, integrative social control was used to reduce disruption and to bring the client back into the organizations' routines for more treatment. Pharmacological interventions were prime examples. If a client was disruptive, staff would attempt—after defusing any immediate situations—to make certain the client was taking medication as prescribed. Long-acting, injectable forms of medication were often preferred by staff, as they rendered compliance less of an issue. If the client was taking medication, staff might attempt changes in form or dosage. Staff would also try psycho-educational or (more rarely) psychotherapeutic interventions. If these interventions did not work in preventing further severe infractions, the extreme response was hospitalization or inpatient drug and alcohol treatment, during which staff expected intensive treatment to stabilize the client to the point that he or she could return to the organization.

The case of Riaan, a client at Urban, was a clear example of this type of informal labeling. With perpetual disruptions, such as yelling with no one in her immediate presence, fighting with other clients, threatening violence, refusing services, and many others, Riaan constantly attracted the attention of workers. Workers informally framed her problems, as they did in her official documentation also, as symptoms of mental illness, saying that her behavior resulted from her "responding to internal stimuli" (field notes). For instance, Riaan was involuntarily hospitalized numerous times for her violent and threatening behavior. However, the organization continued to provide housing and other services to her. As one worker, Steve, put it, "This is the person that we are supposed to most strongly embrace, you know. This is an individual that we need to aggressively continue to work with because, you know, this is somebody who used to fall through the cracks. . . . Just because they are a difficult person to work with doesn't mean that we shut the door [to] her from services" (interview). Interventions with clients such as these were done to "stabilize" them and have them return to receive services from the organization in the community. Nevertheless, these interventions were clearly instances of social control, as the following extended excerpt from field notes regarding Riaan illustrates:

> Steve says she's been making some vague threats. They're getting ready to get things under way [for an involuntary hospital admission]. Steve has already filled out the petition. Wanda, the psychiatric nurse, says that she hates to do it. She says studies have shown that involuntary hospitalization leads to PTSD [post-traumatic stress disorder]. I ask her what led to [the need to hospitalize Riaan], and she says that Riaan was saying that "she was going to get some knives and stab everyone here. That's enough," she says, as if trying to convince herself. "That's enough." Steve calls the police department, asking for the "CIT" [Crisis Intervention Team], the team that deals with psychiatric hospitalizations. Neither the dispatcher nor the dispatcher's supervisor, which Steve asked for, had heard of the team, so they end up dispatching some regular officers. Carla says that the last time they called, the officers were kind of jerks, so that's why they wanted the CIT team.
>
> Steve waits by the door. I wait by Steve. Riaan walks by us and says what sounds like, "White boy, I'll stab that bitch in his face." It takes about 9 or 10 minutes for the officer to show up. . . . A female officer comes, and Steve briefs her. The officer asks how she's doing now, and Steve says "Now she's calm, but she's up and down," motioning up and down. Steve says that it's probably crack-involved—she's probably high. The officer says they see this all the time at the first of the month, when people get their checks. Steve asks if they see extra problems when it's hot outside (today the forecast is ninety-five degrees). The officer says

"Oh yeah. It's a proven fact—full moon, hot weather, first of the month."
Steve says, "Today's a full moon, hot weather, *and* the first of the month."
The officer replies, "Yeah. It should be fun." She's called for backup,
since Steve says that it's hard to predict how Riaan will react to the
police presence. The female officer said that she wanted to wait for the
backup because, "If she just sees *me*," she may still want to put up a fight.
She thinks Riaan probably wouldn't if she sees all of them. While waiting for backup several Urban workers come in and out. Taylor, another
worker at Urban, comes to the foyer. Steve tells him what's going on.
Taylor says "Ohhhh," nodding with an understanding tone. Steve says,
"Yeah, everybody's saying, 'Ohhhh.'" Steve says, "Yeah, I'm pretty sure
I'm not making a mistake on this one. She's not redirectible." . . . Four
more officers, all male, show up. From her reaction, I surmise that the
female officer wasn't expecting this many. The female officer briefs the
others and Steve asks who he should give the petition to. The female
takes it. They all go in.

Riaan's on the phone, and they all wait nearby. Riaan stops talking on
the phone for a minute, and asks, "Who you looking for, Steve?" Steve
tells her that they want to talk to her when she's done on the phone. She
asks why. Steve says she doesn't appear to be "doing too well lately."
She stays on the phone and tells the person on the other end what's
going on. The police officers state numerous times throughout the incident that they're not taking her to jail, but rather to get "an assessment."
Steve also uses this phrase. She says, "For what? I ain't done nothing."
She tells the person on the other end, "They fitting to lock me up in
the hospital 'cause they say I'm talking to myself. I ain't done a damn
thing." She says, "I ain't going to no hospital. You can't make me." She
asks the person on the other end, "Can you make them leave me alone?"
The female officer says, "We can do this the easy way or the hard way."

Riaan says repeatedly that she isn't going and that she hasn't done
anything. She asks Steve who's decision it was to do this. He says "It was
a team decision." She asks him "Can you tell me everybody who decided
this?" He says it was he, Wanda, and "the team. We contacted the people
at your residence, too." The officers do not have to restrain Riaan. She
walks with them toward the door, though she obviously doesn't want to.
Riaan talks louder. "You can't do this. . . . This is ILLEGAL!" The female
officer breaks out the handcuffs. Riaan says, "I'm going. I'm going." The
officer says, "I don't believe you." She says Riaan might try to get away.

Riaan gets loud again. "I'm going to court with this. I'm taking you to court. You can't do this. This is against the LAW!" They head out into the hallway, and Riaan, now in a loud but pleading tone, says "One of you all's got to go with me. One of you all's got to go with me! I can't go there on my OWN!" Steve tells her he will notify her team. He turns to come back in. His group on the other side of the building is twenty minutes overdue to start. He looks at me, visibly drained, and lets out a huge sigh. He starts gathering people up for the group as the police take Riaan out of the building.

Riaan's behavior was no doubt seen as disruptive and was thus subject to control, despite her objections. Although the force with which Riaan was removed from the organization was firm, one can note the compassion the workers showed for her in their requesting the CIT team. Their interactions with her were not judgmental. The ultimate goal was to have her return to the organization after treatment in the hospital, albeit in a more compliant, stable state. Within a few weeks after this incident, Riaan came back to the day program and was allowed back in without a problem.

At Suburban, though the level and type of disruption presented by Riaan was rarely seen, client disruption in terms of more mundane things was more common. One client, Janice, regularly appeared to have trouble concentrating, laughing when no one else was laughing and whispering and mumbling when no one was around. However, these relatively benign problems eventually turned much more serious, and she engaged in "sexually inappropriate" behaviors in public. She was hospitalized several times within a few-month period (though primarily by her family, not by the organization). Workers described her as "out of it" and discussed that her drug "cocktail" might need to be changed. When Janice was admitted to the hospital, her worker, Nicole, wanted to go and see her. However, Janice refused to sign a release allowing Nicole to visit. Nicole was angry, but she quelled some of the anger by viewing the behavior through the informal label of severe mental illness, explaining, "That's the paranoia" (field notes). Though Janice was a potential disruptive presence, and appeared to be attempting to sever the therapeutic relationship, Nicole and Suburban (as well as Janice's family) worked to maintain it, using integrative social control. Janice eventually left the hospital and rejoined the program at Suburban.

Conclusion

Labels are a way we organize our daily lives. This is especially true in bureaucratic organizations. It turns out that—despite the cultural prominence of the

DSM and its official diagnoses of mental illness—official labels of mental illness are of limited clinical use in the daily management of community mental health care organizations for the chronically mentally ill. Official labels of mental illness, in their justification for "medical necessity" for services and their role in triggering Medicaid reimbursement, demonstrate their tie to demands for bureaucratic accountability. These demands render them too tenuous to really guide workers' management of day-to-day organizational life. Thus, staff use informal labels to retain a space for the implementation of the clinical-professional logic and to organize their work experience. To maintain order, staff use social control, but the nature and aims of that social control vary depending on how clients are informally labeled.

In chapter 4 I delve more deeply into the issue of client empowerment, examining the ways staff members work pragmatically to decide how and when clients will have their say in what happens to them.

Chapter 4

Empowerment Practice, Practical Empowerment

[An administrator] may identify people with special [mental health] needs in the community, but also they [those potential clients] have a connection [to an influential person] that we want to nurture for [Wellness, the parent organization], separate and apart from the client or potential client. . . . [Staff at Suburban] don't like to be put in that position all that much. . . . And you can't separate out what should be done with the [client] from . . . what [has to] be done for this [client] because the influential person wants it done. And that's the most unfortunate thing. A lot of the things are good ideas, and should be done. And to some extent, you know, [Wellness] gets to tell [Suburban] how to use resources. Therefore . . . to some extent, if that's how they want the resources to be directed, those [clients] are going to get a little more. But it muddles what is clinically healthy, what is clinically a good idea. . . . You can't change people no matter how much resources you put into them until they're ready, until they want to.

—interview with worker at Suburban

[Jade, the business manager,] says that productivity is going to be more and more of a focus for the [organization, including the day program]. She says there are two parts to productivity: 1) is to make sure they [provide services to] everyone who is [already] there, and 2) is bringing more [clients] in. [There is a discussion of using a point system to reward clients with gift certificates for going to groups. Jeanette, a worker at a

residential program at Urban, is at the meeting and talks of their experience with a similar system there.] . . . Jeanette says it never really worked
at the other program. They gave points for going to groups and doing
chores. She says they "couldn't sustain it." She says they gave out five
hundred dollars in McDonald's certificates in one month. She says they
talked about it: they're giving money to do something, "incentivizing"
behavior, but there's no "removal," which I take to mean transference of
incentive from the [gift certificate] to the inherent value of the practice
itself. She says what they should be doing is trying to make the groups
more attractive to the clients. . . . Jeanette said what they [at Urban's day
program] did was "genius" with the raffle, in finding a way to get people
more incentivized without increasing payout [that is, giving tickets for a
raffle drawing for a reward, rather than giving actual rewards for engaging in behaviors].

—field notes from a day program business meeting at Urban

The two vignettes above highlight how client preferences were key concerns
in the work staff members at Urban and Suburban did with clients. They also
illustrate that other forces shaped how workers attended to those client preferences. In this chapter, we focus on two components of the empowerment
logic, *self-determination* and *provision of resources,* as workers attempted to
implement them within the organizational context (versus broader empowerment in the clients' lives outside the organizations). We do this for a couple of
reasons. First, self-determination inside the organization was viewed by staff
as necessary preparation for broader self-determination outside the bounds of
the facility. If a client could deal successfully with autonomy within the organization, that was a signal he or she was ready for autonomy in the outside
community. Similarly, the channeling of major resources to clients could signal
that the organization saw the client as "ready" to take a major step forward
in broader self-determination. The second, methodological reason to focus on
intra-organizational empowerment is that it was the most evident kind, given
the methods used in this study.

The empowerment logic received widespread rhetorical endorsement in the
mental health system, but there was not a great deal of concrete institutionalization of the logic in the regulations governing Urban and Suburban, leaving
workers frustrated by the ambiguity. In addition, other competing factors were
much more palpable. Frontline implementation of the empowerment logic—that

is, *empowerment practice*—was constrained both by stratification among clients and by institutional fragmentation. In the face of these constraints, workers developed feasible strategies to reconcile the competing demands and still help to empower clients through their work—they crafted a *practical empowerment.*

An Ambiguous Logic

Ambiguity is a pervasive feature of organizations (March and Olsen 1976). The exact goals toward which organizations and their employees should be working are often either unclear or multiple and conflicting. Policies guiding practice are frequently vague about details—perhaps intentionally (Baier, March, and Saetren 1986). This is particularly the case in the human services, where the "outputs" of the work are human beings, making the effectiveness of technologies applied in the work harder to gauge (Hasenfeld 2010a; Lipsky 1980). Even when efforts to implement a logic are not beset by the influence other conflicting logics, the ambiguity of a logic itself can raise issues. At Urban and Suburban, this was the case for workers trying to implement the empowerment logic.

Though some general, abstract principles could be found in the empowerment logic—and were strongly endorsed—there was debate and ambiguity about how to translate those abstractions into practice. For instance, though client self-determination in treatment was a principle receiving strong rhetorical endorsement, exactly who determined under what circumstances the client was able to exercise that participation, and about what issues, was less clear.

Frontline workers in both organizations found the empowerment logic somewhat troubling. They realized (and often shared) the strong normative endorsement of the logic, and the expectation that it would be implemented, but they also experienced ambiguity about exactly how to do so. Because of this, they hoped for some guidance from their organization's administration—though they claimed such direction was lacking. For example, at Suburban, a manager discussed the ambiguous definition of recovery (that organization's iteration of the empowerment logic) regarding client work crews. Crews were made up of clients who, supervised by a staff member, completed tasks around the building, such as filling vending machines, without receiving pay. The underlying goal was for clients' service on crews to teach them work skills and discipline. The manager reported hearing through the grapevine that some within Wellness did not view these crews as recovery-oriented:

> *Manager:*   And I practically picked myself off the floor and said, "It's one of the most recovery-oriented things that [this organization] does."

> *KD*: [Do you think that the administration at Wellness is] going to say crews aren't recovery?
>
> *Manager*: No. See, that's the thing. People are not going to say that. That's—it would be helpful. (interview)

Even though the manager wholeheartedly thought crews were recovery-oriented practice, he said he would abide by guidelines that said the opposite—if such guidelines existed. But they did not. The manager said that, instead of the administration clearly laying out what is and is not recovery-oriented, opinions circulated indirectly, and the management and workers at Suburban were left with different viewpoints and no clear parameters for practice. "And so we're allowed to say we're all recovery-oriented and have diametrically opposed stances on something as concrete as crew" (interview). Similarly, a manager noted in an interview that, although Wellness embraced recovery, the "vision" of what exactly that meant and how to implement it was very "ambiguous" (interview).

At Urban, there was considerable lack of clarity among staff about the details of the harm-reduction approach, Urban's iteration of the empowerment logic, in many everyday situations. Some of this ambiguity surrounded considerations of whether particular actions, on balance, increased or decreased harm for clients. One manager at Urban, for example, talked about debates regarding whether giving clients with substance abuse problems less control over their money fit with harm reduction:

> A lot of [workers] say, "Oh that's not really part of the *harm-reduction model*," you know. "It is their money and they can actually do whatever they want to do with it," and everything else. And I can understand that, but I also think that people need to get out of their comfort zone a little bit more. . . . I think one way to sort of challenge that is to, instead of giving a guy four hundred dollars, or if he's asking for five hundred dollars or two hundred dollars, special request, to not give him the two hundred dollars but to actually give him thirty dollars each week, or something, as opposed to giving him a lot of money. Because that way, *you're reducing his harm,* I guess. You're prolonging the amount of time people get high, but you're also *reducing the amount of harm* that you can potentially do with a larger amount of money, whether he's buying too much or taking too many drugs at the same time. When I've kind of talked about that in the past, some people are on board with that, they think that's a good idea, and that has been done with some clients. (interview; emphasis added)

There was also frequent discussion of how and when to advocate for clients to reduce their harm. Some workers felt that in trying to reduce client harm, the organization too often shielded the clients from the "natural consequences" of their behaviors, preventing them from experiencing the negative effects of their decisions and behaviors. One worker, Ariana, voiced this perspective using the example of housing. She said, "We don't practice harm reduction like it's supposed to be practiced. There is supposed to be accountability. . . . Natural consequences are supposed to occur." She said if someone was evicted from their apartment, "We find them other housing the same day" (field notes). The implication here is that reducing harm (and empowering client choice) through quickly helping clients obtain new housing in a particular circumstance might increase harm to (or disempower) clients long term by reducing the likelihood they would change their behaviors. Ambiguity also attended weighing options in cases where reducing one client's harm could impede meeting the needs of the wider clientele or organization. As was the case with Suburban and recovery, these sources of ambiguity at Urban lined up with larger debates surrounding harm reduction.

Attempting to address such ambiguity in his "practical guide" for empowering people with severe mental illness, Donald Linhorst (2006) outlines several ways mental health workers can help clients be empowered within the organizational context. On an individual level, they can do so by providing clients with housing and employment services and by actively involving clients in their own treatment planning. Moving up a level, Linhorst argues that incorporating clients into organizational decision-making and hiring clients as peer service providers can also be empowering for clients.

A couple of these strategies were mandated for Urban and Suburban. The major national accrediting organization for both Urban and Suburban, the Commission on the Accreditation of Rehabilitation Facilities (CARF), required that both organizations have personalized treatment plans (PTPs), which formally involved clients in determining the goals and means of their treatment. CARF also required client councils, venues through which clients could have input into organizational operation. Moreover, Wellness administered surveys to clients to gauge their satisfaction in different areas, citing it as another official way they solicited client feedback. Similarly, Urban had clients fill out a form titled *What I Want Urban to Help Me With* at first contact with the organization, and occasionally afterward.

Despite having these official means of empowering clients, ambiguity regarding empowerment practice persisted. One effect of this was that staff members were afforded some discretion in how they implemented the empowerment logic with clients. The lack of detail in empowerment regulation allowed variation in how the two organizations implemented those guidelines that did exist. For instance, although both Urban and Suburban both had client councils, they operated very differently at the two organizations. The council at Urban, which met monthly, consisted of a prosumer worker and sometimes other workers disseminating information about program issues to clients and giving them an opportunity to ask questions and give feedback. Informal polls might be taken of those clients present to gauge their viewpoints, with voting usually organized by staff. One example was a vote taken on whether, in extending the hours of the day program, clients preferred the program to open an hour earlier or to stay open an hour later. At Suburban, on the other hand, the client council met weekly and elected officers on an annual basis. Ostensibly, the council had considerable decision-making potential. Clients could bring grievances to the council to be forwarded to the attention of the program director. They also had a budget to spend on activities and could plan parties and other outings. In addition, if its members saw fit, the council could propose changes to program operation. In practice, the council participated mostly in planning activities. In most cases, if staff disagreed with the client council's decisions, the workers could rather easily reject and overturn them.

This example highlights that, although officially incorporating clients in organizational decision-making through a client council, providers retained discretion regarding this type of formal empowerment, which allowed variation between programs and the ability to limit the amount of input clients had. Although both sites were meeting formal environmental demands regarding empowerment practice, there was "ceremonial" adherence to these requirements (Meyer and Rowan 1977), and they had limited impact on the daily practice of empowerment. Analyzing only official empowerment practices would therefore give inadequate attention to what the client and the worker bring to interactions in terms of their own concerns, resources, and conflicts. It overlooked the numerous mundane interactions that take place within organizations between clients and workers, many outside of formal settings. For instance, in the bureaucratically and clinically ideal organization, every interaction between a client and a worker is tied to the personalized treatment plan. The reality I observed was that, outside the formal treatment plan reviews, the PTP was rarely discussed in worker-client interactions. The many interactions clients and workers have in *both* formal and informal frontline mental health care settings are all opportunities to implement or not to implement the empowerment logic.

Constraint in Frontline Empowerment Practice

Even though the ambiguous, limited nature of empowerment regulation opened up room for discretion, there were two major types of restrictions on empowerment practice. These restrictions affected which clients were empowered and which were not. First, some clients had resources that allowed them to impose constraints on empowerment practice. Second, the logic of bureaucratic accountability, with its much more concrete demands on worker practice, at times conflicted with the implementation of the empowerment logic, leading to institutional fragmentation.

Client Status

One set of constraints was rooted in the power balance of the worker-client relationship. Staff members at Urban and Suburban were clients' routes to a wide range of resources. The organizations could connect clients to housing, employment, food, a place to socialize, and assistance in obtaining and managing government benefits. The more resources to which the organization could connect a given client, the more the client was at the mercy of the organization to do what he or she needed to do in order to obtain those resources. Clients did not all want the same things from the programs, however, nor did they all have the same level of need. If clients could access many resources through other means, staff had less leverage over them (Peyrot 1985). These clients could opt out of organizational rules and routines more easily without as much to fear as other clients—they had less to lose.

For staff members, handling the exceptions presented by these less-dependent clients took more of their time and energy. Rather than relying on well-established modes of operating, with these clients workers more often had to craft novel responses to problems and requests and devote more time in meetings dealing with the clients. Handling these clients could also create problems by having effects on other clients, such as when peers realized that a client was being given attention or exceptions that they were not. For workers trying to implement the empowerment logic, these clients could shift staff priorities, using their less-dependent position to divert resources from others. Frequently, these dynamics resulted in these clients having more self-determination within the organization.

At Suburban, a number of clients came from relatively wealthy backgrounds. Some of these were "private pay" clients, having part or all of their care paid for out-of-pocket by their families instead of relying solely on Medicaid, HUD (the US Department of Housing and Urban Development), or other public funds. Importantly, in bypassing this public money, these clients were not subject to some bureaucratic rules and procedures that many other clients were. The distinction between private-pay clients and others was evident to other clients in the organization. For instance, when I took a tour of Suburban's residence given by a client living there, we passed the bedroom of another client. The tour guide made a point to state, "He has a private-pay room, so he can smoke in the house" (field notes). Other residents were forced to go to the back porch of the house to smoke. More broadly, workers described allowing clients from wealthy families to do much more of what they wanted to do in the organization. One worker's comment regarding one of these clients, though blunt, captured the common viewpoint among staff: "Basically, whatever she wants, you know, we're gonna make certain this works—period" (interview).

In addition to clients with financial resources, there were a number of clients with personal connections to administrators in Wellness, Suburban's parent organization, or to other people important to those administrators. In these cases, the clients were dubbed "VIPs," "Very Important People referrals," and they were to be given "special" attention. Some of these clients were the same ones with wealthy families, as some "development"-oriented administrators made a point to cultivate relationships with these families. Clients might also have entered the administrators' radar through their mental health consumer activism or connections to state mental health authorities—not all connections overlapped with financial resources. Others might simply be friends, acquaintances, or other relations of administrators' own families. However they distinguished themselves, these clients were often treated differently than other clients. These clients and their families were not to be dealt with through simple routine interactions. Interactions with them were to be given careful consideration by workers, and the clients themselves often realized this. Thus, through contacting administrators directly or through having their network members do so for them, they learned that they could receive special treatment and have accommodations made for them.

The special accommodations and administrator micromanaging could extend into any aspect of care. For example, one client was the daughter of a board member of Wellness, and workers reported that the parent criticized the care the client received, calling for changes (field notes). Unlike many other parents, however, this parent was in a position to have much of what was called for implemented. One special accommodation that was commonly made for these types of clients was for them to receive vocational services without receiving the other mental health services the program offered, even if staff felt those services were indicated for the client. One client, who was active in the mental health consumers movement and who had connections to state mental health authorities, regularly dealt with issues he felt were not being handled to his satisfaction by threatening staff. One staff member recounted the client asking questions such as "Do I have to go a step higher?"—that is, threatening to take the issue to administrators at Wellness (field notes). Workers saw the stakes as high in these situations: as one staff member explained, "My colleagues . . . are afraid for their jobs" (interview).

Through something similar to a "Matthew effect" (Merton 1968), clients with more wealth or connections were able to garner even more organizational resources and obtain more self-determination within the organization. While many other clients were subject to staff discretion and organizational rules and routines, these "special" clients were able to bend the rules in their favor or disregard them altogether.

It is important to point out, however, that this constraint on worker empowerment practice was not absolute, and often did not depend on the actions of the client himself or herself, but on their network connections. As such, client empowerment based on these connections was fragile, and could at times turn against the client, disempowering them (cf. Peyrot 1985). A worker at Suburban gave an example of how this might occur:

> Frequently, it boils down to . . . the powers-that-be want somebody to get a job. . . . But [the client] is so ill, they don't even talk about jobs. They're not on that page at all. They know that their family wants them to get a job. They know that their family has told that to Wellness, and they're pressured to cooperate in getting a job from all angles. And so, we're not meeting the clinical needs—just rest in a program, learn some coping skills, or you know, whatever, whatever it is—but we're right away focused on getting a job, when this person doesn't have any interest in work. (interview)

Here, although the client did not want to work and was clinically judged by staff as severely limited in *ability* to work, their family wanted them to do so. Because the family member was the one with influence at the organization, pursuing work was what happened. The client's self-determination was undermined; the client was disempowered. However, note that in either case, it was not the workers at Suburban determining what happened; they were forced to go along with the network connection. So, their implementation of the empowerment logic was not theirs (or the client's) to determine—their discretion was undermined. This was in part made possible by the fact that how to implement the empowerment logic was not well defined, which allowed concerns for financial stability and political influence to structure worker-client interaction regarding empowerment.

The clients at Urban lacked the resources and political connections of the clients at Suburban. Stratification and differences in empowerment among the clients was therefore based on different criteria at Urban than at Suburban. The most empowered among the clients at this site generally possessed characteristics that enabled them to function successfully in the context of homelessness, substance abuse, and sometimes a criminal background. Although severity of mental illness (in terms of both diagnosis and severity of symptoms) was one consideration, I will focus on a few more social qualities here.

One of these characteristics was success in street hustling, "indefatigable and creative attempts . . . to find work, make a buck, and make ends meet" (Venkatesh 2006:17–18). Some activities, like selling socks or magazines, were "underground" simply because the income was not reported to the government, but others, such as panhandling, drug dealing, and burglary were more problematic. In his study of St. Elizabeth's hospital, Erving Goffman (1961) found that patients who were "con-wise" "often showed very rapidly that they knew how to work the system" (214). I found that, at and around Urban, successfully living homeless (a position that nearly all clients at Urban had occupied at some point) or spending an extensive amount of time on the street, especially for active substance abusers, often involved developing skills to persuade and manipulate others. Many clients had learned these skills by necessity.

Within the organization, differences in ability to hustle were evident in everyday interactions between workers and clients and between clients themselves. Often these interactions involved access to basic necessities the organization offered, such as food, gift certificates to restaurants, and toiletries. At times, clients attempted to obtain resources from workers personally, such as workers' personal money or old clothes that workers gave to clients on occasion. At other times, clients might try to persuade a worker to have their meeting at a local restaurant or café, where they could have the worker buy them food or drink. Clients also tried to hustle each other for food or a hit of a drug. An example of the difference between those who could hustle and those less successful can be seen in the two following field note excerpts dealing with lunch in the day program. In the first, Ferdinand, a client successful at hustling, manages to get seconds at lunch. In the second, George, a less adept hustler, is caught trying to obtain extra food and is denied.

> Ferdinand tries to hustle Foster, who's talking about if there will be seconds. . . . [Ferdinand says,] "I didn't even get firsts." I saw him eating and served him myself [but I do not say anything]. Foster tries to jump him in [the lunch line], but Ferdinand says, "No, that's all right. You all go ahead." He ends up getting served again. [Another client,] Darnelle, sitting there witnessing things, laughs. (field notes)

> George is in line, and Steve says to him. "George, you've already eaten." George replies, "I know, but I'm still hungry." Steve shakes his head and motions for him to get out of line. George complies. (field notes)

Those clients best able to hustle staff ended up directing more organizational resources to themselves and could "work the system" of organizational rules and routines to empower themselves.

Most clients at Urban did not work in the traditional labor force, instead relying on various forms of public assistance, but some did receive income through involvement in various endeavors in the underground economy. A segment of clients worked as day laborers or sold newspapers or socks, while others engaged in drug dealing, sex work, or money lending. To the degree that the income was consistent or considerable, these clients relied less on what the organization offered in terms of basic necessities. Though they might take advantage of the organization's food, activities, or shelter, clients with alternative means to obtain resources (unlike other clients) could opt out, choosing to ignore what was required to obtain resources from Urban: following organizational rules and routines. They could also make life difficult for workers through engaging other clients in their disruption of those rules and routines.

A problem for staff was that these alternative sources of income kept clients away from services that Urban offered, services directed to empower clients to work toward the larger goals they might have—or that workers might have for them. These clients might also engage in activities (for money) that severely increased risks to themselves and others (for instance, sex work or dealing drugs), which undercut many larger goals that workers were trying to help the clients achieve; client independence was ideally a goal of both clients and workers, but taking part in the underground economy was not included in treatment plans.

So, although hustling and working "off the books" might meet clients' needs, it did not generally count as meeting treatment goals. Further, engaging in these endeavors made the organization's offerings less attractive. The basic services that Urban used to "engage" clients in care were less of a draw if they could be obtained through other means. Thus, these clients in many cases maintained the lowest level of participation in services that they could, just enough for staff to have them sign their forms documenting participation. "They need them signatures," as Walter, a client who sold newspapers and worked as a day laborer, said in an interview, speaking of Urban's day program. Staff members were helping him apply for Social Security benefits and provided him with housing, but his off-the-books jobs allowed him to avoid coming to the day program most days and to limit contact with the organization generally.

Some clients working in the underground economy caused troubles for workers' implementation of empowerment through their effect on other clients. A couple of clients in particular were brought up in these discussions. One was a client who dealt drugs—including to other clients. This client knew when other clients received their benefits checks and was sure to appear at the day program on those days. When he left the program on these days, anywhere from five to ten other clients left with him. One worker observed that the dealing client had better attendance in his dealing "groups" than the staff member could garner in his own treatment groups (field notes). From the perspective of the empowerment logic, staff members were ambivalent about the client's drug dealing. As one staff member put it at a day program meeting, they needed to consider that he was a nonviolent drug dealer in a harm reduction–focused program, and workers needed to "decide what that means" (field notes). On the one hand, his product was thought to be not overly adulterated with dangerous chemicals, and he was not known to be violent to other clients. So, his selling could be seen as reducing those risks for his customers and giving them what they appeared to want. On the other hand, many staff—especially case management team workers—felt that the client's dealing was undercutting the goals they or their clients—his customers—had been working toward, such as reducing drug use or better money management. They saw this client's dealing as pure exploitation. For a long time, no staff directly observed the sales, but the client was eventually caught dealing in the program's bathroom and was barred for a time. Later, he was arrested on the street for dealing, and he was convinced one of Urban's staff had reported him to the police (field notes).

Similarly, another client, a former drug dealer and gang member who said he no longer dealt, frequently lent money to a few other clients, charging them

100 percent interest (per month). It was unclear how much staff knew about this practice, but they did seem to group that client in their minds with the drug-dealing client and other former prison inmates. The mixed feelings and ambivalence regarding those clients was captured by one staff member's comment, as recorded in my notes: "She says that she doesn't doubt that [these clients] could have problems and need medication, but this isn't the place where they should be treated." They were seen as unsuitable for the organization's services (Peyrot 1982; Roth 1972). One worker cited, as an example of the drug-dealing client's exploitation of the organization and its services, that he was able to pay two thousand dollars to bail himself out of jail and still came for free lunch and services as if he were extremely poor.

As a critical complication, self-determination was seen as central to the empowerment logic, but the details of how that translated to everyday practice were not clear. In general, staff agreed that even though many clients at Urban were understood to be using illegal drugs and were going to spend much of their money on drug use, obtaining drugs or money for drugs from other clients was not acceptable. Moreover, through drug dealing and usury, some clients were channeling many of the resources the organization gave to other clients to themselves, thus creating a hierarchy of empowerment.

To summarize, these mental health care organizations were not the only component of clients' lives. Clients differed in their activities, networks, and other available resources outside the organizations. Thus, workers were not able to routinize and treat all clients the same, and differences in client's histories, relationships, and resources were consequential for client empowerment. Two of the key components of the empowerment logic, client self-determination and provision of resources, were stratified among clients in ways that workers found difficult to manage and over which they had limited control.

Institutional Fragmentation

A second constraint facing how workers implemented the empowerment logic was rooted in another logic with much firmer institutionalization: the logic of bureaucratic accountability. In the organizations I studied, the empowerment logic was not translated into many clear rules or regulations governing staff's work with clients. In such situations, if other environmental demands are more clearly translated into organizational structure and bureaucracy, they will have more influence on organizational behavior (cf. Bryson 2005). Celeste Watkins-Hayes (2009) found that in the welfare departments she studied, there were two different models of a good worker: the "social worker," who connected clients to services, helped them achieve independence, and changed clients' lives, and the "efficiency engineer," who efficiently processed paperwork and closely monitored client eligibility and rule compliance. Whereas a great deal of rhetoric was devoted to the former, much greater weight was ultimately given to the latter in worker evaluations. Similarly, I found that at both Urban and Suburban, the bureaucratic logic imposed much firmer controls on workers' behaviors than the empowerment logic, delivering strict sanctions for not following rules and regulations associated with it. Organizations could lose funding and workers could lose their jobs. Although workers might feel they *should* help clients become empowered, the consequences for not doing so were often unclear and rarely severe. At the same time, staff found themselves *required* to implement the bureaucratic logic, which sometimes clearly conflicted with the impetus to act on the empowerment logic. In these instances of institutional fragmentation, workers were forced to make a choice between two different standards (Sosin 2010), with the clearer imperatives and sanctions of the bureaucratic logic more frequently winning out. The two components of the logic of bureaucratic accountability most evident here were documentation and productivity.

The push for documentation meant that staff members constantly monitored, tracked, and made formal note of client activities, especially their own interactions with or about clients. Because of the potential for auditor review of these bureaucratic notes and threats to funding if they were not completed correctly, the organizations instituted internal review of documentation practices in order to catch mistakes before they were caught by outsiders. The organizations argued that detailed documentation was also in the best clinical interest of the clients, but the financial importance was much more frequently mentioned. Workers felt these pressures and acted on them in their interactions with clients. This could lead to conflicts when clients did not want to participate in the bureaucratic processes. So, one act of self-determination clients were *not* empowered to make if they wanted to receive services was choosing not to participate in organizational bureaucracy. Clients' signatures were often required for many types of documentation, which could cause problems if they did not want to give them or were illiterate. However, if the provider was going to receive funding for serving the clients, clients needed to sign. In these circumstances the bureaucratic logic was determined to be more important to implement than the empowerment logic. A manager from Urban demonstrated this fragmentation and its consequences. She explained how client noncompliance with paperwork could lead the organization to be unwilling to continue providing rent subsidies to them when they were kicked out of their housing:

KD: Are there times you don't give them another subsidy?

Manager: There are many times. . . . Like, from the business aspect, [we have to take] into consideration, you know, did—is this going to be a problem with our funder? Is this going to possibly jeopardize our grant? Because for HUD-funded programs, there are required pieces of paperwork that we have to have from the participants on an annual basis. . . . If that particular person has not been compliant with their HUD paperwork, that could actually put us into jeopardy with our funder. (interview)

So, if the client wanted housing, which is one of the top services clients at Urban sought, he or she must complete the paperwork.

The pressure to participate in these processes increased after changes to state policy and organizational software. Though they might not understand why, clients did notice the changes. For instance, one client at Suburban, Shara, noted one day in leaving the workshop portion of the program that clients now had to sign out whenever they left. She said she did not know why. "We didn't use to have to" (field notes).

Another component of the bureaucratic logic, productivity, brought the importance of finances even more to the forefront of worker activities. Not only were workers judged regarding how meticulously they documented what they themselves and their clients did, but they were also evaluated by how much of their work was billable for the organization. So seeing more clients, for longer periods of time, and engaging with them in activities for which funders paid or reimbursed the organizations, was increasingly important for workers. With this imperative from the bureaucratic logic ever-present in workers' minds, the concerns of the empowerment logic were often pushed out or outweighed.

One example of this was that, at both organizations, there was a move to restrict worker interactions and activities with clients to those that were billable. Not all discussions workers might have with clients were about mental health, substance abuse, housing, or other billable topics. If they were not, staff members were not supposed to bill for them. Similarly, as Urban business manager Jade explained, "Transportation is not a billable activity. . . . If you're in the car with the client and having conversation with them, then you can bill that as a sort of activity. But when I get on the train or the bus or in the van, and I drive to a participant's home and I'm by myself, that—that is not billable" (interview). Thus, staff members were pushed to minimize or alter these activities and increase activities that were billable. This could lead to fragmentation with the empowerment logic when clients wanted to engage in interactions or activities that were not billable.

This conflict, between client self-determination and productivity, was one of the issues most starkly noted by workers at Suburban. Given complete self-determination within the organization, clients might spend quite a bit of time engaged in activities for which the organization could not bill—client empowerment might not be good business (cf. Townsend 1998). Workers were receiving two strong but conflicting messages. Catherine, a staff member at Suburban, captured the contradiction while discussing the problem of clients sleeping in the day program: "We get in trouble if we tell clients not to sleep, but then if they sleep we can't bill for them and then we get in trouble because our hours aren't high enough" (interview). Problems also arose with clients who did not attend consistently, making it difficult for their workers to produce sufficient number of billable hours. Staff could not easily impose sanctions on clients for not attending (because of the recovery approach), but were low on billable hours because their clients were choosing not to come regularly.

Similar issues were present at Urban. Many clients would receive a periodic check from their benefits account and disappear for several days—presumably abusing drugs. Other clients would schedule appointments with staff and then not show up for the appointments. Staff frequently attributed this to the problems facing Urban's clientele—homelessness, severe mental illness, substance abuse—which had led to their being rejected by many other service providers. If a client broke an appointment, staff members were stuck frantically trying to find another client to engage with so they did not lose billable time. Even when clients did meet with them, however, the meetings were often very short if left up to the client. Often, the client simply wanted to obtain their benefits check or lunch and immediately leave. However, if the staff member could keep the client around for just eight minutes, they could legitimately bill for a quarter hour of time.

A common problem for both organizations dealt with recreation activities. A major motivating force for clients to engage in services generally, or in recreation activities in particular, was food. One worker at Suburban put it bluntly: "The only reason why these folks are gonna move is if you tell them there's a meal at the end of the day. Period. And we [staff] all know that" (interview). Frequently, the first thing clients mentioned when asked about any activity outside the organization that had involved eating was the food. Both organizations frowned on food being the sum total of community recreation activities, however, in part because of audit issues. Similarly, clients at both organizations enjoyed going to the movies, but the organizations could not bill for time spent in the movie. So, even though clients wanted going to the movies as an activity, it was restricted as an offering because staff could not bill for it.

Workers were clearly being pulled in different directions. They felt the push to enact the empowerment logic but received relatively little concrete guidance on how to do so. On the other hand, in many situations they received rather strict guidelines about productivity and revenue generation. The reason for these concrete bureaucratic guidelines was that these organizations found it difficult to keep the lights on if they did not force their workers to engage in revenue-generating activities. In turn, workers threatened their own jobs if they attempted to implement the empowerment logic in ways that conflicted with the bureaucratic logic. Thus, we have a quintessential instance of institutional fragmentation.

Practical Empowerment: Workers' Adaptive Strategies

The constraints just outlined ensured resource flows for the organizations. Individually wealthy or powerful individuals could have a great deal of influence over the fate of nonprofit organizations. Their demands, and the concrete practices associated with the logic of bureaucratic accountability, took precedence over empowerment concerns. Workers restricted client self-determination and were limited in controlling how resources were channeled to some clients. However, workers developed some strategies that attempted to salvage some implementation of the empowerment logic while working within the constraints they faced.

No staff member let clients completely dictate goals and treatment, nor did any staff member deny client decision-making under every circumstance. Strategies used by workers varied depending on the conditions of particular situations and their view of specific clients. The barriers of time and resources made it impractical to allow client choice for every client at all times. Thus staff members developed a strategy of *allocating choice*, deciding that some situations and some clients were more appropriate for autonomy in treatment and others less so. This involved determining both how autonomy would affect the client and the amount of work produced by granting autonomy. If self-determination in a situation was likely to lead to the client putting him- or herself in imminent danger or would lead to a lot of hassle or "cleanup" work for the staff member, the worker might attempt to prevent the client from exercising choice. Clients who were seen as symptomatic were less likely to have strict social control applied to them. At other times, if a client was seen as capable and independent, workers might rank interactions with them low priority because other clients were seen as having more pressing needs. This could conflict with the client's desire to meet with workers for, among other things, the benefits of companionship. For instance, as I shadowed Stacy, a case management worker, we visited Fontina, a woman that Stacy described as one of these independent clients. Because of this, there was a gap between what Fontina wanted from services and what the staff was willing to offer her. Fontina said that I should come and visit her at her apartment. "They're too busy," she said, motioning to Stacy. After Stacy dropped Fontina off at her house, she explained that, because Fontina is so high-functioning, workers found it hard to have social visits and "entertain her," because they had so many other (presumably more pressing) things to do. So, she said, they could not sit with Fontina "for an hour," and they at times "put her off." According to Stacy, when Fontina herself had things to do, she would say she did not want to have a visit (field notes).

When dealing with constraints based on client status, allocating choice could involve bowing to pressure from VIPs to go against clients' wishes—for example, pursuing employment that a client did not want. It could also involve refusing to bow to such pressure and denying demands from the wealthy or connected. As mentioned, however, workers feared this would result in their losing their jobs. For "con-wise" clients at Urban, this strategy manifested in workers' decisions to bar clients for behavior with which they did not agree, regardless of whether it reduced the risk to the client or other clients.

Allocating choice commonly involved fragmentation between the competing demands of the empowerment logic and the bureaucratic logic. If clients caused problems for the providers in ways that prevented them from obtaining funding, they might sacrifice client self-determination in order to bring in resources. Recall, for instance, that not completing required paperwork could lead to a client being cut off from services. Not meeting minimum participation thresholds could also lead to problems for some clients (though not others), threatening their ability to receive services in the organization. Barry, a worker at Suburban, described an interaction he had with the mother of Barnabas, a client on Barry's caseload who lived at the organization's residence. Barnabas was spending extended periods of time away from both the residence and the day program, making it difficult to provide services—and to bill for provided services. Barry said he told Barnabas's mom that Barnabas's not being at the house was a problem because they needed to pay for the bed, and "rent ain't going to cover it." Barry said that a manager, surprised, asked him, "You told her that?" He said the manager nodded in agreement and said, "Yeah." Barry said if Barnabas was away from both the house and the day program, then Suburban was not receiving anything for having him enrolled. "From Barnabas's perspective," Barry said, "maybe this [the organization's services] isn't what he needs. If it *is* working for him, then we need to find out how to make it work for *us*." Barry said Barnabas needed to attend house meetings and to participate in a couple of groups in the day program. According to Barry, the difference between Barnabas, on the one hand, and other clients at the residence who did not spend sufficient time at either the day program or at the house, on the other, "is about seven figures"—millions in family wealth (field notes). Because the other clients' families have connections or contribute resources directly to the organization, they are allowed to remain with the organization without facilitating other resource flows through billable activities. So even within strategy of allocating choice, there were limits to worker's actions. Without such wealth or connections, Barnabas was not afforded such self-determination.

For those clients determined inappropriate for choice, staff members were at times outright directive, basically ordering them to do what workers wanted them to do. For example, one day at Suburban, Serena, a mousy client who frequently missed groups and did not attend the program very regularly, was confronted by her worker, Nicole. As I walked in the room, Nicole was raising her voice at Serena. Serena said that she did not know how she was getting home that day, so she was calling someone to try to figure that out. Nicole said, sternly, "Now's not the time to find that out, when you have class." Serena stopped, and Nicole persisted, "Go on." Serena stood up and left, presumably to go to class (field notes).

At both organizations, workers at times used another method to restrict client choice: leverage. Staff's control over resources clients wanted allowed them to use coercive techniques to limit the choices available to clients (Appelbaum and Redlich 2006; Monahan et al. 2005; Robbins et al. 2006). Housing and money were common points of leverage. At Urban, workers held the clients' benefit checks until clients interacted with them for what staff saw as sufficient time, often a minimum billable unit. Once the client interacted for an acceptable period, the worker would hand over the check. As stated earlier, however, some clients were less dependent on the organizations for such resources, so the method was not uniformly effective.

Working with clients was not necessarily a "binary" event between choice and coercion. Even while presenting a range of options to clients—a key part of the self-determination component of empowerment practice—workers could nonetheless influence client choice (Angell, Mahoney, and Martinez 2006; Peyrot 1985). At Urban and Suburban, this involved workers actually engaging with clients to elicit goals and desires but presenting the choices as not all equally attractive. I refer to this strategy as *steering choice*.[1] A form of this strategy was an integral part of motivational interviewing (Miller and Rollnick 2002), a mode of working with clients that was formally endorsed by both organizations. Motivational interviewing involves using clients' own ambivalence about behaviors to motivate change. One reason for the attractiveness of steering choice was that it enabled staff to say that clients freely chose to make the choices staff wanted them to make; from the staff viewpoint, clients then practiced self-determination *and* made the right choice. The important variables in this strategy were the number of choices presented as valid and the degree of balance used in weighing the costs and benefits of each choice. Workers did not always represent all choices or describe those choices they did present as equally acceptable.[2] Catherine's description of using the strategy was typical: "I try to show [clients] both sides of the equation, but I try—I don't know. I get my side of the equation to a look little better" (interview).[3] This strategy was also evident in the explanation one worker at Urban, Ivan, gave of his interaction with a client, George, regarding the client's medication, and the reaction of other workers to the interaction. Ivan said that George asked if he had to take his medication. Ivan replied, "First, you're right, you don't have to take them, but here are the consequences of not taking them." He said he told George that his symptoms would worsen, he noted the pain caused by crack addiction, and he said he reminded George that the last few times he went off his medication, he was thrown in jail and suffered other negative consequences. Ivan said that a nurse and a worker from the day program became very angry with Ivan for his response. They said that he should have just told George the consequences, but not confirmed that he did not have to take his medication (field notes). Ivan acknowledged George's ability to choose whether he would take his medication. However, he also explained all the negative effects of doing so. His stance on the medication was clear. He did not, for example, discuss all the positives of not taking medication as well. Nevertheless, his coworkers thought he should have steered harder in his interaction with George.

Administration at both organizations endorsed a form of this strategy in dealing with the fragmentation between the empowerment logic and the bureaucratic logic. At times, the response to problems with client attendance might be allocating choice. Another proposed solution at both organizations, though, was to "motivate" clients to participate without forcing them to do so. If they could convince clients to participate in billable activities, then they could have the best of both worlds. At Suburban, this was exemplified in how the program dealt with clients sitting idly in the lounge area, which was not billable. The staff was held accountable if clients did so, and the guidance they received was that they had to motivate clients to do other things—not force them to do so. For instance, one day at Suburban, Glenda tried to round up people for an outdoor gardening group, despite the overcast sky and misting rain. Two clients, Janice and Barney, were sitting in the lounge area, as was I. Glenda asked Janice if she wanted to go with the group, and Janice immediately stood and joined Glenda. Barney was playing solitaire. Glenda asked Barney if he wanted to go. He looked at her as if he was gauging if he had to go, hesitantly standing up. Glenda, perhaps noticing his ambivalence, then said, "It's up to you." Barney immediately sat back down and said he did not want to go (field notes). Through her nondirective engagement, Glenda was able to prevent one of the clients from sitting in the lounge but not the other. However, she would be able to say that she attempted to call on both the empowerment logic and the bureaucratic logic. At Urban the strategy could be seen in adjustments to the token economy at the day program, as illustrated in the second vignette that began this chapter. Clients received coupons for attending groups, which could be used to obtain lunch. But soon after I began my fieldwork, it was determined that people should not be kept from food because they did not attend groups. So a change was made that the coupons would be for a raffle instead, where items such as gift certificates, toiletries, and hats were given out. By using such strategies, the coercive aspect of worker-client relations was (ostensibly) removed, but the incentive to engage in billable activities was kept—once again implementing both the empowerment and bureaucratic logics and incorporating incentives for both workers and clients to engage in the behaviors (cf. Handler 1996; Linhorst 2006).

Steering choice was used frequently to deal with the conflict of empowerment/bureaucratic institutional fragmentation, but I have little evidence of it being used for constraints based on client status. On one hand, this strategy might appear to be a great way to defuse conflict with a wealthy or connected client, avoiding repercussions through having the client choose to comply. On the other hand, these clients' privileged status made them less likely candidates for this type of strategy. Wealthy and powerful network connections served to broaden the options open to clients, so that they were less bound by any options presented to them by lower-level workers. Further, for clients adept at hustling, their skill at persuading others probably rendered them less susceptible to many persuasive attempts used by workers. Finally, for both types of clients, their wider range of resources outside the organizations made it less likely for them to rely on workers to solve many of their problems in the first place.

Conclusion

Although the empowerment logic in its varied forms received rhetorical support in the mental health care system and at both organizations, it was far from clear to workers how it was to be implemented. A couple of key constraints limited the amount of discretion workers had. One was rooted in stratification among clients, which differed at the two organizations. At Suburban, clients with wealth and powerful network connections could have more resources directed toward them and could have more self-determination, beyond or in addition to what workers thought was appropriate. Clients at Urban who were employed in the underground economy or who were "con-wise" could likewise muster more resources and have more self-determination than other clients, undercutting staff's ability to implement the empowerment logic in the ways they best saw fit. The other major constraint came from the logic of bureaucratic accountability, with its much more concrete institutionalization. The strongly enforced guidelines limited the role of the empowerment logic, leading to institutional fragmentation. Staff adapted to these constraints in a few ways, though not all strategies worked equally well for the different constraints. One strategy was allocating choice, determining when and how clients could be given self-determination. Another strategy was steering choice, attempting to influence clients to freely choose options that staff members wanted them to make, thereby preserving aspects of both logics.

This chapter demonstrates once again the centrality of concerns about financial stability in the nonprofit service sector, and how these concerns affect day-to-day practice. The experience of Suburban's wealthy clients and VIPs shows that these organizations are constantly looking for new forms of revenue and stability (Pfeffer and Salancik 2003 [1978]). Since government and nonprofit granting organizations are major sources of funds, the bureaucratic logic becomes dominant. However, other revenue sources (here, wealthy family members) or powerful network connections (VIPs) can have more idiosyncratic demands that do not fit neatly within that logic. Nevertheless, as has been demonstrated in other social service fields such as child protective services (Smith and Donovan 2003) and welfare benefits workers (Watkins-Hayes 2009), both

Urban and Suburban were forced to balance the demands of the bureaucratic logic against other demands. Workers ended up adhering closely to the bureaucratic logic, and their desire to implement the empowerment logic was pushed to secondary status.

Chapter 5

The Realities of Community Integration

[I talk with Marin, a manager at Suburban, near the end of my fieldwork. We discuss the sheltered workshop, and how the parent organization is shutting it down.] I ask if the clients are all going to participate in the supported employment program and work in the community. He says he doesn't know, but looks doubtful. He says, "Some people worked here because they didn't want to work competitively." He says [Wellness, Suburban's parent organization,] has been wanting to get rid of the workshops for a long time. I ask him what the reasoning they gave was. He says, "It isn't compatible with current and coming models of care, which I agree with. But, [pause] then you're taking away a choice."

[On another day, we talk again.] Marin says [one client, Dick,] got a job through the supported employment department in Wellness and worked as a bagger in a grocery store or something like that. [Dick] decided, however, that what was involved was not worth the amount of pay he was getting, so he quit and decided just to do the workshop here. Now that it's closing down, he has no plans to try to obtain other competitive employment options. Marin says that out of the [about two dozen] clients who would work in the workshop any given week, four to six of them are being "motivated" now to pursue competitive employment by the closing of the workshop.

—field notes, Suburban

Connor says [that after a recent backslide in treatment] he's been hanging out on the street a lot. He said that's a problem, though, because when he hangs out on the street, he wants to drink, and when he drinks, he wants to "play games," and some of the games he plays can get him put in jail. Ricky [another client and Connor's friend] asks him what he means by "playing games." Connor says, "You know how we play games." Ricky says he does, but some others may not, so he asks on their behalf. Connor says "we" [he and Ricky] grew up on the street, and things that other people are scared of, ["we"] do: getting high/drunk, robbery, assault, soliciting "hos." He said he realizes that it was stressful, everything he was doing [before the setback]: going to groups, staying away from his friends, going to anger management classes, going home and going to bed. He said it's very hard to do that when you are trying not to drink, too. He says that drinking is bad, but "not drinking is even worse."

—field notes, substance abuse group, Urban

Unlike state mental hospitals, community mental health care organizations have semi-permeable boundaries with the communities that surround them. Though confidentiality regulations assured that not just anyone could enter Urban or Suburban, clients could and did spend time in the surrounding community, especially those at Urban. The amount of time spent in the community and how far into the community they traveled varied greatly, however. Consistent with the community logic, workers generally saw the ultimate ideal goal of the services they provided as reducing client dependence on the organization and helping them live in the surrounding community (Bond 2004; Gulcur 2007). As the vignettes above demonstrate, however, the external community held risks for clients, and not all clients were interested in the degree of independence and integration into the "natural" community that the community logic held as the goal for them. Thus, the empowerment logic could come into conflict with the community logic, revealing a site of institutional fragmentation.

Problematic "Community"

Despite its entrenchment in the mental health services system, the dominant form of the community logic was problematic for a couple of reasons. Both reasons intersected in some way with the logic's uneasy relation to clients' lived experience of community.

Providers' and Clients' Communities

The community logic was firmly institutionalized in the regulatory environment and in the minds of workers at both organizations. One of the key components of the logic is *integration with the natural*, meaning that the client should be integrated into his or her natural environment, which the logic defines as life and social supports outside the organization or other mental health care setting. The client needs some connection to the mental health care organization to receive services, but the level of involvement should be minimal even then, and quickly reduced as much as possible. Although the hope that family members and beneficent community members would care for these clients might not be realized, life in the community is nonetheless held in higher esteem than life in a state hospital. So, one of the foundational goals of any community mental health services personalized treatment plan, including those at both Suburban and Urban, is the "prevention of unnecessary hospitalization." Services and assistance provided to clients were for the purposes of training and development, not simply sustenance. Despite these lofty goals, the community logic did not take into sufficient account how clients actually experienced community, both before and during their involvement at Suburban and Urban.

The logic appeared to assume that before clients became involved with community mental health care organizations, they lacked community ties. In the past, when most people with severe, persistent mental illness spent years in state hospitals and lacked any sustained contact with the outside world, such assumptions might have been justified. However, though some clients from both Urban and Suburban were referred to the organizations through state hospitals, many others were not: family, nursing facilities/institutes for mental disease (IMDs) (which, though similar to hospitals in many ways, were not generally as physically isolated as many hospitals were), and job services organizations were other sources of referrals. At Urban, many clients reported becoming involved with the organization through other people they knew on the street or through Urban's own homeless outreach efforts, not through other organizations. So, many clients already were involved in communities, and many maintained these ties even after they became involved with the organizations.

Once clients began receiving services from Urban and Suburban, they encountered the push for integration into the external community. Again, however, this push was based in a logic that overlooked the communities into which many clients were already integrated. Although the quality of the relationships associated with these communities was often questioned by both workers and clients, they were quite consequential for organizations' efforts at community integration for clients. At Urban, many clients had relationships with other people on the streets surrounding the organization who were not clients there. The basis of these relationships ranged from socializing to sharing and exchanging drugs. There was usually a group of clients and non-clients milling about the front entrance to the building throughout the day while the various programs of the organization operated. This could cause problems when clients worked to physically integrate into the community and maintain their progress outside the organization's walls: they literally had to pass through their old "community" on a daily basis. In the second introductory vignette that begins this chapter, Connor, a client at Urban, pointed out that he had not coped well with a setback he had experienced. This was at least in part due to the physical proximity of his community. Every time he entered or exited Urban's building, he encountered those who tempted him to engage in what he and staff saw as problematic behaviors that could undercut his progress.

At Suburban, clients often experienced community through relationships with staff and patients at IMDs, if they lived there, or with their family members, with whom many lived or still had some relationship. In some rarer cases, families had regular contact with clients and were seen as playing a relatively positive, supportive role for them. They could provide material and emotional support. More commonly, however, if family was involved, their relationships with clients were seen as problematic by the family member, the client, or the organization. In some cases the family was seen by the organization as partially responsible for the client's condition and as an impediment to their recovery. This was the case for one client at Suburban, Casey, who was removed from his family as a child due to abuse and spent a good deal of his childhood in residential treatment. During my time there, he had reestablished contact with his mother's family and was visiting on weekends, much to the chagrin of his worker, Catherine. She explained:

> Casey will be with his family on the weekends, and they will be telling him how terrible we are and we are stealing his money and he should come live him them and everything will be great and there would be no rules. And they're not gonna be abusing him anymore. It wasn't their fault. And [children services] is crazy. It's [children services] fault. They took him away. And this kid, he is finally getting a relationship back with his family. And he was dying for their love and acceptance. And then he comes [to the program] and he's conflicted and brings these things to me and he tells me. And I know what they are doing but I can't sit there and say, "Casey, they are doing this and this and this," you know? He says,

"What should I do? Should I go there? Should I quit Wellness and live with them?" . . . They really make him feel like crap about it. So it is like clockwork. By Friday he's awesome and then he goes with them on the weekend and then in one day he is a wreck again. (interview)

Other families were felt to be overly involved in clients' lives, calling clients' workplaces numerous times a day to speak with clients' supervisors, or telephoning their landlords (field notes). On occasion, clients themselves saw the family members as hampering their abilities to improve their lives. Connor described how after he was released from prison, he initially lived with his sister. However, the drug dealing and chaos of her home led him to choose homelessness rather stay there: "A lot of bad things were going on in my sister's house. She—my nieces are grown up; they got boyfriends that sell drugs. And the police kept coming there and kept coming there, so I couldn't take that, you know—the police, the drugs, and all of that that was going on. So I went into a shelter" (interview).

Why did these "other" communities matter? Because clients' involvement with them affected their integration into "the community" as the community logic envisioned it. Clients had spent large chunks, if not the entirety, of their lives involved with these communities. Some clients at Suburban had never moved from their parents' homes. Clients at Urban frequently had spent four or five years homeless. Clients at both organizations had spent years living in nursing facilities or IMDs, and at Suburban, many still lived in them. Life in these institutions and groups could greatly pattern how clients thought and behaved, developing into what Pierre Bourdieu (1977) referred to as "habitus." The habitus (and there were many, depending on the group or community) clients developed in these communities remained even after clients left them. The "transposability" of clients' dispositions was a hurdle to staff and the community logic's ideal community integration.

For those who had lived for long periods in nursing facilities, IMDs, or with their families, a common result was a habitus characterized by isolation and passivity, which workers found difficult to overcome. With clients having nearly all aspects of their lives determined for them in these settings, including such things as basic money management, leisure activities, meals, and chores, it was difficult for staff to help clients take the initiative to determine what they wanted to do. This was not only because what they would choose might not be considered appropriate by staff, but also because many clients were just not used to making decisions for themselves; family members or IMD staff had made those decisions for them for a long time. Suburban worker Catherine recounted that Casey regularly asked before using the bathroom when he first joined the organization (interview). Nicole, also at Suburban, described more generally how the independent living skills clients developed at the organization were undercut by their roles at their parents' homes or at IMDs: "Well I think . . . sometimes the clients come here and they're learning skills to be independent and then they go home and they go back to assuming this role of dependency" (interview).

The durability of these dispositions was a formidable obstacle for workers. Because providers generally worked to integrate clients into the geographic community in which the organization was located, if clients' friendship groups were likewise located in the area, they would naturally gravitate toward them. However, these communities lacked many of the qualities organizations attempted to work with clients to attain: sobriety and stability in terms of symptoms, residence, and finances, for example. As Connor put it, people in the organization monitor clients' health and well-being, providing them with what they need. On the street, which is where he spent time outside the organization, "There's no thought on anything that would benefit you. Everything is what will destroy you" (interview). Nevertheless, given the choice between associating with strangers or with those they knew, who might be bad for them, many clients chose the latter for the sake of familiarity.

Groups and situations that even so much as resembled clients' former communities could cause problems, as the clients' ingrained reactions were often different from what staff—or even clients themselves—desired. Wherever they were, clients were drawn to similar groups, characterized by similar ways of thinking and behaving. Changing to a different way of living, as staff tried to work with them to do through community integration, was very difficult for them. For example, one client at Suburban, Phillip, had a history of drug use. Working with Suburban, he obtained a job and eventually an independent apartment. However, he later was kicked out of his apartment because, as he put it, he "got mixed up with the wrong people," a group of drug users where he lived (field notes). A worker at Urban, Jonas, described a client who had been homeless for years. Though Urban obtained housing for him, he would not immediately stay in it:

> When he first came in, he looked at the housing a few times, refused it, and eventually he agreed to move into the backyard in the building. So he continued sleeping outside just behind the building even though there was a warm room inside where the rain didn't reach. And for a month or two he stayed still sleeping outside. He then moved under the

back staircase, still outside, and when he moved inside recently, he slept on the floor, and I'm not sure if he's moved to the bed yet. (interview)

For this client who had become accustomed to living in the elements, it took months of work and small steps for him to transition to living in the increased safety and shelter of an apartment or a soft bed (cf. Duneier and Carter 1999). So, work with clients on community integration had to contend not only with their mental health and substance abuse problems but also with their former communities and the dispositions they had cultivated through those communities.

Internal versus External Communities

There were additional issues with the communities that workers *did* attempt to integrate clients into that rendered community integration problematic. Many surrounded an important distinction that was often not fully considered in community integration efforts: the difference between external and internal integration. In their study of "community-based sheltered care" facilities in California, Steven Segal and Uri Aviram (1978) argue that external and internal social integration consisted of the same components: presence, access, participation, production, and consumption. Internal integration was the degree to which clients were integrated into the mental health services organization's community, whereas external integration was the degree to which clients were integrated into the community outside the organization. Subsequent studies of community mental health have tended to overlook this distinction and the relationship between internal and external integration (Mandiberg 1999). More important here, the conception and implementation of the community logic did not give enough attention to the difference. In its push toward integration with "the natural," the community logic failed to address certain barriers to integration—some of which the organization itself erected—and the attraction of the organization's internal community itself. Both these issues could act against integration into the external community.

First, many of the activities in the community with which organizations engaged clients were not practical for clients to reproduce on their own. Many were cost-prohibitive for them to participate in on any regular basis without the organization's paying. For instance, many of the popular groups at Urban that went "into the community" involved going to cafés and fast-food restaurants, with the organization paying for the food. Though the stores were in the neighborhood, and thus by frequenting them the clients were meeting some goals of community integration, clients could not expect to maintain that community relationship without the providers' support. When they did, as Enis, one client at Urban, did by frequently going on his own to a local café, they could be viewed as irresponsible with their money. A community support worker expressed in a staff meeting how Enis was spending too much of his money at the café, and the worker planned to talk to him about it (field notes). Even public attractions, such as museums, cost money to visit or to arrange transportation to. The organization paid and provided transportation when going as a group. Clients would have to pay themselves if they went on their own—no simple task.

Another major problem with this ideal external community was that it was not always welcoming to clients. Urban's buildings were in an area where there were many social and mental health service organizations; however, the neighborhood was gentrifying, and as often occurs with the influx of new, wealthier residents (Brown-Saracino 2010), tensions arose between the recent arrivals and those residents receiving human services. Both workers and clients at Urban reported an increased intolerance for Urban's clients. Local stores and restaurants were commonly unwelcoming unless clients were to buy something and often wanted to make sure clients were going to buy something up front. For example, signs at one diner a few blocks from Urban read as follows:

RESTROOM IS FOR *PAYING CUSTOMERS ONLY.*
WE RESERVE THE RIGHT TO REFUSE SERVICE. PAYMENT, IN
ADVANCE MAY BE *REQUIRED* BETWEEN THE HOURS OF
6AM AND 7PM (field notes)

Another chain store required tokens, which were doled out by store staff, to use their restrooms (though this policy was changed near the end of my time there). Those people who had yet to obtain housing said they faced increasing surveillance and hostility from police, who, in turn, were reportedly facing increased complaints from residents. Sometimes locals did not wait for the police to intervene, as the following incident I observed one afternoon illustrates. An apparently homeless man lay/slept in the doorway of an auxiliary entrance to Urban's building. As I walked by, a clean-cut man in a button-down Oxford shirt passed by. He yelled harshly at the sleeping man "Get up!" (field notes). Urban's housing programs were also being "targeted" by those in the neighborhood, who did not like the element they attracted, according to one residential staff member (interview). Even if the clients had housing and a little more income, past experiences of this kind of treatment could leave their mark, leading clients to be reluctant to be present "in the community."

Homelessness and outright hostility from the local community was less an issue at Suburban. In rural and suburban environments, the problem for people with severe mental illness is less homelessness than it is "carlessness" (Floersch 2000) and poverty. Clients' limited access to reliable transportation was a source of client—and worker—problems. Even though they might have housing, many clients at Suburban did not live in the town where the provider was located, but rather in an adjacent town. Thus, being transported to "community" destinations on their own was difficult. Even though local establishments lacked the unfriendly signs of those near Urban, the expectation of payment or purchase—the need to be transported there by public transportation or taxi and to purchase something to stay there—was still understood by clients and raised barriers to their frequenting them. Many clients chose to stay at their residences, socializing with their parents or other IMD residents. If the IMD happened to be on a busy street, then clients might congregate in front of the building, smoking and watching passers-by, as was the case at one such facility where many clients that attended Suburban lived. Those who lived with their parents might accompany their parents on their outings and social events.

In light of these barriers to participation, one can understand why clients would have trouble with the organizations' dominant conception of community integration, instead opting for the familiar. One additional option was *internal* integration into the community built within the organizations themselves, which had a host of benefits for clients rarely found in the external communities. However, these internal communities also had several problems that prevented them from being ideal for clients.

Several aspects of the organizations' communities made them very attractive options for clients. First, organizations required some clients to be present at the organizations' physical plant for certain periods in order to receive services. Walter, a client at Urban, explained his integration into the organization's community and how his attendance was a requirement:

I just sit [in the program] and chill, like you see me [outside], smoke a cigarette, socialize, then come on back [in the building] and sometimes I help them cook, this and that, attend a group or something, make phone calls. . . . What I was hearing is that you are supposed to attend a couple of meetings a week because that is good, you know, for their, for their books, and let them know what is going on, you know what I mean? Because, like, them people, they come down and check and they go, "Okay, what is up? Why are these people not attending any of these groups? You all is not doing your job." They got to have so many signatures, to let them know what is going on. They come and check. "What is you all doing? Are you all really putting pressure on these people?" (interview)

At another point, Walter explained that he would probably spend his time elsewhere if he was not required to spend time at the program. The requirement facilitated his integration. Suburban emphasized the requirement more than Urban, even more so after receiving guidance from the state department of mental health. As a manager explained at a staff meeting, a representative said that psychosocial rehabilitation is meant to be an intensive service, so clients were supposed to be there at least eight hours a week. If, after being at the program for six to eight weeks, they were not meeting the requirement, the manager said they could begin to "ask if this is the right place for you," and would have the option to "boot" the client from the program (field notes). Though the threats attached to noncompliance with this requirement often appeared idle, there was an expectation that most non-residential clients would attend the day program at both sites. Although simply being present somewhere does not in itself constitute integration into a community, being increasingly involved can make that presence much more enjoyable, providing an incentive for clients to become integrated into the organizational community.

Another benefit of these internal communities was that they were generally more accepting and welcoming to clients than the external community. Not only did the organizations provide a space where one could sit and relax, but they also provided resources—both material and social—to clients, all without necessarily requiring payment from service recipients. As Marin, a manager at Suburban, stated it, "For the vast majority [of clients], this is the most resource-filled and nurturing place they have." So clients could obtain free coffee or food (though obtaining food sometimes required chores), friendly interaction, a soft couch or chair to sit in, and other comforts of public spaces. Moreover, the groups and activities available at Urban and Suburban gave the clients an engaging escape from the isolation of their living situations, again, without requiring money. Many clients said one of the best things about attending the organizations was that it was "something to do." Further, unlike in the external community where, if clients were not outright rejected, they nonetheless often experienced the indifference of the general populace, in the providers' facilities, clients encountered staff and other clients who they felt were genuinely concerned about their well-being. As one client at Suburban, Phillip, put it, the people at the organization were "like friends and family" (interview). Even "bad" clients, for whom staff had less tolerance, generally received better treatment in the organizations than that they received in the outside community.

Finally, these organizations provided a safe atmosphere for clients, the kind rarely available in the outside world. They were safe in two ways: First, there was physical safety, in that aggressive incidents were much less frequent and less serious in the organizations than they were outside, because they generally were not tolerated. For homeless clients, the organizations also provided shelter from the elements of nature. Second, there was social safety, in that clients were encouraged to talk openly about potentially stigmatizing and emotionally troubling issues, whereas such types of topics were generally not brought up in conversation in the external community. Moreover, they were allowed to behave in ways unacceptable in the outside world. Talking to people others cannot see, claiming that one is Jesus, or other such behaviors led to social exclusion in everyday life, but not in the organization. This sense of safety was addressed by Connor:

> The people that come here are people that are intimidated by the people in the neighborhood. They feel safer here . . . as a group than [they would] to be the one, the only one [with mental problems] amongst everyone else that are supposed to be "sane," you know what I mean? . . . Here, they have a group and . . . here, they're taken care of. Down in these shelters, I'm telling you, the things that [clients] do here, they wouldn't get away [with] at the shelter. You know what I mean? The guy who's running the shelters would be more belligerent with them. The person that they would make a mistake with would probably try to knock the hell out of them, 'coz they're stupid and bullies, you know. So here, they're safe, you know, they feel that safety. Plus, they feel that "Here, I can get away with more here than I can get away with out there." So they're safe here, they feel safe here. (interview)

The benefits clients obtained by integrating into the internal community of the organizations also came with generally lower demands placed on them. As mentioned, unlike at many places outside the facility walls, at Urban and Suburban clients generally did not have to pay for services, because the state or their families were paying on their behalf.[1] Further, clients did not have to contribute to organizational operation through either active participation or labor in order to receive the benefits, unlike in the wider society. However, we will see below that the expectations tied to benefits actually varied depending on how the staff labeled clients.

Given these benefits of integrating into the internal community of the organizations, it may not be surprising that some clients chose this community to the exclusion of external integration. However, the organizations themselves did not encourage this, and at times actively fought it, which could lead to conflict. The conflict involved not only differing conceptions of community but also clashing views on client empowerment.

Institutional Fragmentation

There was a palpable push for integration into the external community in the community logic. What was less clear was exactly how fast the push should occur. Recall that the original introduction of the Community Support Program stated that services should be of "indefinite duration" (Turner and TenHoor 1978). However, both Urban and Suburban worked to reduce the amount of time clients spent in the organization's care. Changes in state policy were aimed at increasing the delivery of services in the clients' "natural" setting—that is, outside the organization's walls. Both organizations had to provide the majority of services (60 percent) outside the facility's physical plant. As a manager at Suburban put it, "There is no longer a thing called a day program" (field notes). Many of the services that were provided through the day program were now to move outside the providers' walls. The point was to focus on services instead of programs—not giving clients a *place to go*, pushing them and assisting them to find places and relationships in the community.

The effect of this push was much more notable at Suburban, where there had already been less focus on engagement and more on independence and integration into the community. Many of the workers who had previously provided psychosocial rehabilitation groups in the organization became community support workers who worked with clients individually outside the organization to pursue their goals. A manager said that the state had communicated to Wellness that the parent organization should "get rid of the real estate" and just have "roaming workers" that worked with mental health clients in the community (field notes). At Urban, there were definite changes in services—for example, assertive community treatment teams were transformed into community support teams—but there was also a concerted (and largely successful) effort to do things as they had always been done. Importantly, there was no noticeable reduction in the volume of clients who spent time in the organization's building during the day—in fact, there was a move to increase the number. At least some of Urban's difference from Suburban in this respect was due to the different role each site played in the community logic. Urban focused on engagement, connecting previously unserved clients to services and trying to keep them connected, whereas Suburban was geared more toward helping clients achieve independence. Nevertheless, at a training dealing with implementing state policy changes, a manager at Urban said that the state wanted the staff there working with clients toward independence *in the community* as much as possible, "instead of creating chronic PSR clients," that is, instead of clients receiving services in the organization long term (field notes).

This push toward the external community continued a decades-long movement of freeing clients from a life confined to mental institutions. Part of the attraction of the *Olmstead v. L.C.* decision was that it built on this trend. In the decision, the US Supreme Court ruled that mental health clients cannot be held in state institutions against their will if they could be adequately cared for in the community. However, even with community services, clients could nonetheless spend the majority of their day behind the walls of a mental health services provider. State regulators encouraged providers to facilitate further independence, but the push appeared to be based on an assumption that my research revealed as problematic—that all clients *wanted* that movement toward independence and integration into "the natural."

In their impressive book, Russell Schutt and Stephen Goldfinger (2011) describe an empowerment-oriented housing demonstration program for people with severe mental illness that aimed to help its clients be completely self-sufficient after eighteen months. Though each residence would initially be fully staffed, the plan was for staff to work with clients to build their confidence and skills, with the residences completely client-run by the end of the program. Despite the plans, however, none of the residences entirely did away with staff during the program. As the authors explain, there was "variable interest [on the part of] tenants in acquiring more responsibility. Tenants did not uniformly or consistently favor reducing staff control, and many tried to avoid taking on more responsibility" (215). Although the program staff was willing (however begrudgingly) to turn over the houses to the clients, not all clients wanted that all the time. This illustrates a major issue with the type of push toward external integration and independence I described at Urban and Suburban. Such efforts apparently assume that clients themselves hold those goals, which was not, in fact, always the case. Many clients at Urban and Suburban would *choose dependence* on the organizations, resisting efforts toward independence and integration into the outside world. The provider became a tool the client could use to avoid making tough decisions or to evade acting on choices they had already made, as workers stepped in to set boundaries and make choices for the client.

Clients would choose dependence when they felt unable to control their behaviors due to symptoms of mental illness or addiction, or when they had a habitus developed through many years in institutions. For example, Darnell, a client at Urban, talked about how having the organization as his payee (the entity that received his benefits checks from the government), which removed his own control over his money, was good for him. He said it reduced his harm from drug use: "Well, being a part of the program is harm reduction in itself, letting them be my payee. Letting them have to pay the rent, you know. Because, other than that I get carried away, I get obsessed, and won't nothing matter but the next one, the next high" (interview). Even one of the most vocal client activists at Suburban, Daniel, chose a mental health services organization (though not Suburban) for his payee, because he felt his mental illness could lead him to go on spending sprees (interview).

For clients who chose dependence, being pushed toward independence could be distressing. For example, Grace, a client at Suburban, became quite upset one day when a manager made the comment "Clients need to not rely on staff so damn much" during an all-program community meeting. Later she explained, crying, why she was upset. She said that day was the first day she had not felt tired in a very long time. Her doctor had changed her medications, which allowed her to finally have a good night's sleep. Thus, maybe she could do more. She said it was very hard to be heavily involved in the program when you are tired all the time. Not everyone has the energy (field notes). Her response was not an isolated incident, and a few months later she addressed it in a meeting of the client council at the program (of which she was an elected member). "Not everything is independent. [Staff] should stop harping on it and be happy they [clients] have as much independence as they have. You have to give these people what they want! Their independence may be sitting there!" (field notes). Clients experienced a number of fears related to this strategy. For example, some clients feared working because they thought the additional income might lead to them losing their Social Security benefits. Moreover, if they reported improvements in their illness, they would be expected to take on increasing responsibilities. This also meant being held more responsible for their actions.

Recall that a key component to the empowerment logic is client self-determination, that is, clients being experts in their own lives and care. This principle held that they should be active participants in their own treatment planning. Thus, if they felt they did not want to be independent, from the empowerment perspective, they should have been allowed to remain dependent on the organization until such time when they felt they wanted to be more independent. However, with the community logic solidly pushing clients out of the organization and into the external community, client self-determination to choose dependence was undercut. The empowerment logic was somewhat ambiguous regarding the details of client empowerment, and mental health system regulation did not contain all that many regulations covering client empowerment; despite this, staff felt (and were told) they *should* empower clients. The community logic, on the other hand, was tightly tied to funding: if organizations did not have at least 60 percent of their services outside of the organization, they risked losing funding for community support services. Further, the community logic was firmly entrenched in workers' minds—staff assumed clients were to work toward integration into the community as the end goal. Though not immediately obvious, the community logic and the empowerment logic clashed when clients chose dependence, and staff had to decide how to proceed in the face of this institutional fragmentation. Though it was a delicate balancing act, in most cases, the community logic won out.

Among workers, even the most vocal advocates of client self-determination appeared to have a problem with clients choosing dependence. Their endorsement of clients making their own decisions clashed with the embeddedness of the community logic in their minds. Flint, a manager at Urban, described his view on the issue in an interview:

Well, the way I think . . . ideally is that we're trying to help people live without the mental health system . . . to live or at least to live more fully and completely in the community. And, I mean, one thing I think our mental health system is really good at is creating mental health patients, and, and, I think, of sort of fostering the dependency on the mental health system. Now there's a lot of ways I think you can spin that. . . . [One is to say,] "Well, well that's, that's, for those people the mental health system *is* their community and that's, that's the only place they can get community and what's wrong with that? And then, because of who they are and how they function and because of the rest of the society, the only place that people with mental illness or substance use problems can go to get community is programs. So that's just the way they're going to be. And that, the idea that people are going to be able to live out in the community, I mean it's nice and ideal that, you know, let's get real. It's probably not going to happen." Well, okay, I, I guess that's true. . . . That's not how I think about it, though. I think that well maybe, now mental health services can be *one dimension* of the, of that particular person's life. And let's face it, even with our services people are only here what, a third at most of their life [per day]. I mean they're still, even with us, they're still living their—the majority of their lives—outside of our walls and relationships.

For Flint, as the community logic dictates, the goal is to move out of the organization's internal community into the external community, even if the movement cannot be complete. For him, the system itself has cultivated the dependence that clients now choose to perpetuate. This viewpoint is perhaps how Flint, a steadfast proponent of client self-determination, is able to reconcile the community logic with the empowerment logic: if the system was different, the clients would make different choices.

Along these lines, both organizations worked to nudge clients toward independence and external integration through policies. At Urban, for instance, clients in many of their housing programs had their own leases with the landlords. So, the landlord had to deal with clients directly, forced to seek court approval in order to evict them. Other mental health providers operating in the area held the lease for their clients and made agreements that client residence was on a month-to-month basis, making it much easier for the landlord to kick them out. As an employee at one apartment building pointed out, this type of agreement also made it much easier to have the providers intervene to address landlord's problems with their clients (interview). As mentioned, Suburban's parent organization also eliminated the sheltered workshop at Suburban, even though many clients enjoyed working in that setting and preferred not to enter competitive employment.

Harvey, a worker at Suburban, said he would (gently) push clients who chose to be dependent on the organization to consider integrating more into the external community:

> *KD*: So, what if clients come in and say, "I'm here and I want to be here." Do you really, really, really work with them to [push them into the community]?
>
> *Harvey*: Well, with the clients who do like being here, like, there are some clients here who have been here a number of years. They've wanted to go through the whole level system in which they are not only learning their skills, but for one reason or another, they may not utilize a lot of those skills, but they still like coming here because that's part of their daily routine. That's okay, too. That's also part of recovery.

But working with them about talking through, What are your thoughts about beyond here? When are you going to do that? What is your thinking about life after here?

KD: So what if they decide that they don't want to think about that?

Harvey: Then we just work with them on talking that through, and/or we say, "Okay, we're okay with that," but we just let them really, really brew on it and let them think it through. We're just here, really, at least, I think, this is just me, I think we're here really to assist them with whatever goal or whatever dream, whatever value system that they have that they want to work with. (interview)

Harvey describes a very delicate balancing act in working with clients, one in which he does not allow clients to accept, uncritically, dependence on the organization, but he does respect their right to do so if they actively consider it and decide that is what they want. It is clear that he sees the ultimate goal as greater integration but reconciles that by moving at the clients' own pace.

Attempting to apply the empowerment logic and the community logic to clients, workers did not treat all clients the same or have the same expectations of all clients. The distinctions could be mapped onto the different categories of clients outlined in chapter 3. Staff had fewer expectations for clients informally labeled *symptomatic* to integrate externally than they did for the *good* and the *bad.* The decision of these latter two groups to choose dependence was morally evaluated. Because they were viewed as having the ability to actively pursue external integration, they were expected to do so. However, there was even a distinction in staff's reaction to these two groups, with the good usually receiving a lesser push toward integration than the bad. If a client who was not labeled symptomatic chose relative dependence on the organization, they were less likely to be pushed if they conformed to the rules and routines of the organization than if they were disruptive. Compare Harvey's diplomatic, generalized response above to this more detailed, critical reflection on certain clients within Suburban:

Harvey: Well I—I think for me what I've noticed is that, the word "complacency" seems to come to mind a lot with clients. Some clients just like the status quo. And they don't want to change and they don't want to grow. They don't want to do anything other than stay where they are. That to me indicates someone who doesn't want to use the program. They want to use the system, but not the program. That to me is two different clear, different things. . . .

KD: And what about somebody who uses the system? What does that mean and how does that—?

Harvey: That—that—and this why I struggle with this. I—I struggle because I know that those aren't recovery terms. But I struggle with that because I can clearly tell the difference when somebody wants something . . . just to get what they want, instead of doing the steps it takes to develop those skills in order to obtain those things on their own. A good example of that is there are some clients who live, who are in our [group home] who love to come [to Suburban's day program building] and they want a job, but they don't want to keep the job. They want our bus pass, but they don't want to pay for it. They want to live in the house, but they don't want to pay the bills. They—you know, I mean, so they figured out a way to manipulate. . . . Trust me, in the [time] I've been here, there have been clients who try to manipulate me into doing things for them. And at first I would've—I would've done it and learned from it, but now that I've been here and I've seen that and I've experienced all that, I've made a decision, "No, that's not something I can let you do." (interview)

It is evident from this that Harvey wanted to apply the empowerment logic in its recovery form, respecting client self-determination. But he had a very difficult time doing so when dealing with clients who chose dependency, who he saw as being able to do more. When he felt that capable clients tried to manipulate him and depend on Suburban, he refused to participate.

The effect of informal labels on staff expectations is also illustrated in how staff at Suburban dealt with two different clients, both of whom had official diagnoses involving psychotic symptoms. One client was Kim, who had moved to Suburban's group home after living in an IMD for five years. Overall, staff saw Kim as capable and, in general, ready to move out of the group home to live independently and to hold steady employment. Diagnosed with schizoaffective disorder, Kim seemed to have her symptoms under control. However, she was one of the residents of the group home that Harvey alluded to in his statement quoted above. Staff thought that she had an unnecessary dependence on them for things that she was able to manage on her own. For instance, they said that she would not plan transportation to appointments by public transit, instead waiting until the last minute and then asking staff for help in paying for cab fare. She had reportedly admitted to faking auditory hallucinations because she thought doing so would aid her in avoiding having to go to some therapy appointments. Staff claimed that Kim would pursue employment opportunities and independent housing, and be offered both, but would then "sabotage" both. She quit jobs and turned down housing options.

Staff members were frustrated with the time and energy they invested in helping Kim, only to have her not follow through and manipulate, and so they began to withdraw their supportive services from her. At one staff meeting workers discussed how Kim was offered a job that had a decent wage and benefits, but she was worried about transportation to and from the job and asked for the organization's help. A staff member at the house, Suzanne, said she "put the ownership on her" by telling her that she would have to hold the job for two weeks, arranging her own transportation during that period, before they would assist her (field notes). Similarly, during another staff meeting, a housing staff member said Kim asked if she would go with her to an appointment for a housing provider that had accepted her. The worker said, "No, because she wouldn't take anything they offered" (field notes).

Contrast this with the way staff, in a meeting, discussed another client, Kathy, who was experiencing severe psychotic symptoms. Kathy's psychiatrist, who was not affiliated with Suburban, thought she should obtain a volunteer "job that she doesn't want," according to her worker, Glenda. At the meeting staff recounted her symptoms, including "zoning out," hallucinations, and other psychotic symptoms. Transportation was also an issue. Glenda said she tried to work with Kathy in the past regarding taking public transportation. She said she sat behind Kathy on the bus one time, moving farther and farther away to build Kathy's confidence and comfort, but Kathy finally said no, she didn't want to learn to take the transportation on her own. In the end, the consensus seemed to be that Kathy was not ready at that point to pursue a volunteer position, so her wishes to not pursue it should have been respected. However, a manager also said that they should "set small goals with the client, and deal with the transportation issue" (field notes). Although staff respected her wishes regarding work and transportation, the gentle type of push that Harvey demonstrated was still recommended for her. So firmly entrenched was the community logic in regulation and in workers' minds, that complete lack of effort toward integration was not acceptable even for the symptomatic.[2]

Conclusion

The mental health care system in the United States has come a long way from the days of institutionalization. Care now often happens through organizations firmly embedded in communities, and mental health providers attempt to transition clients to live increasingly in those communities and away from the organizations and their workers. However, clients receiving this care have lives outside these organizations that affect what happens in treatment. They may have strong ties to segments of "the community" that undercut their progress in treatment, such as drug users or family members who foster dependency. Clients may feel stigmatized by their illness or rejected because of their relative poverty, or may feel unsafe in the community, leading them to believe that the best community for them is the community found inside the organization itself. If clients choose dependence on the organization, workers are in somewhat of a bind, because the empowerment logic says they should respect that, whereas the community logic says they should be pushing clients to integrate. Workers thus sorted patients by level of illness (as describe in chapter 3), allowing the sickest to choose dependence (to a degree—though not completely), pushing the least symptomatic to integrate more and judging them if they did not. However, in the broader mental health system, belt-tightening changes in policy from a government worried about budgets is making it less and less possible for clients to remain dependent on organizations, raising questions about what kind of community they will integrate into if they are forced to integrate before they themselves feel they are ready.

Another question raised is the nature of empowerment in these sites of fragmentation. If many clients develop deeply entrenched dispositions through their years of dependence on family or mental health care providers, they are more likely to choose dependence. These dispositions would not easily be changed through providers simply offering choices to clients. Cultivating new dispositions likely would take extensive treatment that at times involved not allowing clients to choose their preferred options. Is it disempowering if the result is a client that felt more comfortable choosing from a wider range of options? For instance, what if coercing clients to spend more time outside the organization led clients to develop more confidence and positive interactions there? They thus would have the ability to base their decisions regarding integration on these new experiences, making it more likely they would *choose* independence from the organization. Were they empowered overall? Such philosophical questions are beyond the scope of this study, but they frequently underlay fragmentation between the empowerment logic and other logics in community care.

Chapter 6

The Right Person for the Job

Fragmentation in Staffing
and Worker-Client Interaction

Two short months into his tenure as an employee in the day program at Urban, Emmanuel Short had already dealt with a number of incidents that even a veteran worker would find notable. He had broken up a fight between two clients, actually grabbing a chair out of the hands of a client who was the size of an NFL lineman—two to three times Emmanuel's own slender size. He had also confronted a client he witnessed selling drugs in the bathroom and was, as a result, threatened by that same client when he left work later that day. Add to these a number of smaller volatile incidents, and Emmanuel had established himself as someone who could handle the tough parts of the job, even though he said he hated to deal with conflict.

Despite this, Emmanuel interacted with clients a bit differently than some other workers did. He was able to develop close relationships with clients, which other workers noticed right away. For instance, he quickly developed a bond with Pharrel, a highly symptomatic client who was a constant source of crisis and disruption for the organization. Emmanuel said he talked with Pharrel in depth one day, helping him to "identify with what is it that's disturbing him and why is it disturbing him and how, if he'd change his perception and accept some things that's happening, and just go through it, his life would change." Emmanuel said one of Pharrel's case managers told him he immediately noticed the effect that talk had on Pharrel: "I don't know what you said to him, but his whole attitude's changed." The case manager told Emmanuel that Pharrel apologized to him for how he had been acting. Another client, Carlton, had likewise formed a special bond with Emmanuel, often seeking him out before others to discuss his mental health and substance abuse issues.

One explanation for Emmanuel's ability to form relationships with some clients can be found in his own background. Not only was Emmanuel Black, like most clients at Urban were—including Pharrel and Carlton—but he also was hired as a "prosumer," having dealt with drug abuse issues and severe mental illness himself. His problems, which had begun early in his college years, had eventually led him to spend time in prison and to experience a brief bout with homelessness. He was court-ordered into a twelve-step-based drug treatment center and into mental health treatment. He obtained employment in the mental health system through that mental health provider, eventually landing a position at Urban. When I met him at Urban, he was still receiving mental health treatment and attended twelve-step meetings daily, having been clean and sober for nearly a decade. Emmanuel framed his work at Urban as sharing his own hard-earned life wisdom with people who were going through what he had gone through in the past. "I believe God gave me a purpose, and my purpose today is to help people who are just like me," he said. "These are people who are *just* like me. I was once just where they are." So in some ways Emmanuel saw his job as an extension of his role as a longtime Alcoholics Anonymous and Narcotics Anonymous member: "sharing experience, strength, and hope," as the saying goes. And the boundary between his life outside the organization and inside the organization was much more fluid than it was for many other workers. For example, Emmanuel's mentorship relationship with Carlton extended outside the organization—he was Carlton's sponsor in a twelve-step program. He also recommended that other clients with free time after Urban's day program closed attend the local twelve-step meeting he started.

This closeness to clients' issues was a means of bonding with clients, but there was a flip side to it. Emmanuel wondered how his coworkers saw him. He said there was a female staff member who used to talk to him frequently and then one day suddenly stopped. He thought maybe she "found something out about" him, perhaps saw him on the department of corrections website. I asked if he was more open with the clients about his life than he was with staff members. He said he was. He said most staff members only see participants' lives from a distance. He said he, on the other hand, had been "right there where they are!" He said he had recently heard staff making fun of a particular client, joking about how the client expressed a desire to commit suicide. Their response stung Emmanuel. He said, "That was me! I tried to commit suicide—a couple of times."

Emmanuel's situation was a common one for a segment of workers at Urban and Suburban. With peer support becoming an increasingly prominent part of contemporary behavioral health services, one finds more and more workers sharing clients' backgrounds and experiences. However, alongside this trend remains the firmly entrenched grip of professionalism. Two logics—the clinical-professional logic and the empowerment logic—shaped both hiring and who was considered a good worker at Urban and Suburban. Those in charge of hiring valued both logics but experienced them as pulling them in different directions, fragmenting their staffing of the organization. The result was groups of workers who interacted with each other and with clients in distinctly different ways, as well as a workforce stratified by clinical credentials and worker backgrounds. The clinical-professional logic was dominant, used to judge and oversee staff members who were hired based on the empowerment logic.

Institutional Fragmentation in Staffing

A battle has been waged throughout the health and human services field over roughly the last half century between the (withering) dominance of service professionals and the (ascendant) movements to give more rights and input to the consumers of services. In the mental health services sector, the shift to a more consumerist orientation has affected both the services offered and the organizations that deliver them. It is not uncommon to see mental health care organizations run by mental health consumers (Clay et al. 2005; McLean 2000; A. Scott 2012). Peer support—people with behavioral health problems helping each other—receives widespread endorsement within the mental health field—at least rhetorically. However, funding streams have not opened to the principle to the same extent mental health discourse has. Researchers and policymakers have lamented the lack of reliable state funding for consumer-run services. Instead, these programs are likely to be funded through grants, a more tenuous source, which threatens the programs' long-term stability (Clay et al. 2005). Practically speaking, what this means is that peer support providers, or prosumers, frequently work in organizations dominated by coworkers who do not share those issues.

Although they work in the same organizations and are even hired by the same people, prosumers and other mental health workers differ in how they see themselves and in how they are seen by those who hire, supervise, and work alongside them. Both types of workers are seen as valuable to the providers, but reasons for each differ. One can detect distinctions between prosumers and more clinically trained workers in both how they are hired and how they carry out their work.

The story of these distinctions is in part the story of two institutional logics in hiring. Although the mental health services field has shifted to incorporate the empowerment logic more fully, the clinical-professional logic has not disappeared. The concerns and imperatives of both are evident throughout mental health care organizations. Thus, those in charge of hiring must consider the concerns of both logics—specifically, they must consider clinical expertise *and* peer support.

Administration at both Urban and Suburban were confronted with regulations that forced them to consider both logics in hiring. Recall that state Medicaid rules classified workers based on experience and clinical credentials, from a Rehabilitation Services Associate (RSA)—requiring no credentials—to a Licensed Practitioner of the Healing Arts (LPHA)—requiring advanced certification/licensure in a clinical field such as psychiatry, psychology, counseling, or nursing. Similarly, regarding the empowerment logic, with new state service definitions, if either organization decided to provide Assertive Community Treatment (ACT) services, each ACT team would have to include one person "in recovery"—a prosumer, in other words. Ultimately, neither organization opted to provide this service. However, Urban provided Community Support Team (CST) services. The CST service definition stated that having a person "in recovery" on the team was "preferred." This gave discretion to the organization, but if the organization was trying to please the state auditor, they would likely feel pressure to have a prosumer on the team and hire accordingly. So, understandably, CSTs at Urban included prosumers.

Much more clearly evident, however, was the value placed by workers themselves on the concerns of *both* the clinical-professional logic and the empowerment logic in staffing. They wanted workers who had extensive clinical training as well as workers who clients could identify with and receive peer support from. They felt they should have staff with good clinical skills and staff who shared the background of clients.

Those in charge of hiring at both organizations expressed the advantages of having people with "good clinical skills." Often this was translated into a desire for those with clinical licensure and educational credentials. For instance, one manager at Suburban, Glenda, discussed how she was pleased with the skills possessed by her current employees: "I feel like the people I supervise now have really good skills. . . . Some of the staff have some really good clinical skills and—and some master's classes in, whatever, theory and all that. So in some ways they can handle a lot more than other people. [They] have been in the field and did behavioral therapy with people. . . . It is really nice when you don't have to explain things about reinforcement modeling and people get that pretty quickly. They can go with that and they understand that there is a purpose to being consistent" (interview). A manager at Urban, Jessica, talked about someone she planned to hire for a position: a woman who just received her master's in psychology from a local school. The education attracted Jessica. She pointed out the value the organization was making in the hire, as the candidate was educationally overqualified: "So I've got someone with a master's degree in a position that . . . someone straight out of undergraduate is technically eligible for" (interview).

Alongside this desire to have clinically credentialed workers, there was also a desire to have workers who reflected the background of clients. In line with the traditional definition of "prosumer"—a professional in human services who is (or has been) a consumer of the services provided—one set of criteria often considered was whether prospective employees themselves had been consumers of mental health and substance abuse services. Along these lines, Suburban's parent organization had an officially "affirmative" hiring policy, wherein consumers of mental health services received preference in obtaining jobs with the organization. At Urban, though the preference was not ensconced in official policy, several individual managers indicated wanting prosumers for particular positions—often for part-time positions.

Personal experience with mental illness or substance abuse was not the only background characteristic outside of clinical credentials that those hiring saw as valuable. Managers also attempted to match clients and workers based on demographic characteristics such as race, ethnicity, gender, and age. Jessica's comments illustrate this broader perspective on hiring from the empowerment logic: "I know that clients have said, you know, 'Ah, these White people they don't care' or whatever, when they perceive that something's, you know, not fair or whatever. And I think that that highlights why it's important to have, to the greatest extent possible, a multicultural team and diverse in terms of ethnic or racial background, life experience, education . . . [and] nationality" (interview). Though less explicitly stated—perhaps because of the relatively less diverse clientele[1]—the tendency to try to match client and staff background was noticeable at Suburban. For instance, a Black worker at the organization remarked out loud in a staff meeting in which new clients were being assigned to workers that "all the dark-skinned" clients were being assigned to him (field notes).

Those in charge of hiring at Urban and Suburban said they found it difficult at times to fulfill the criteria of one logic or the other in any given hire. Unlike the "professional ex" path described by J. D. Brown (1991), many of the prosumer workers I encountered did not pursue "credentialization," making it difficult to satisfy both the empowerment logic and the clinical-professional logic in one hire. When these and other uncredentialed workers did pursue education, it was often in a field unrelated to mental health services. One prosumer at Urban said her dream job would be a chef. An uncredentialed worker at Suburban had a degree in the arts and worked part time in the arts field in addition to his full-time job at Suburban. Another uncredentialed worker at Suburban was likewise pursuing a degree in the arts in evening classes. Nevertheless, a minority of prosumers and other uncredentialed workers did pursue education in mental health–related fields. These included two prosumers at Urban without college degrees pursuing certifications in psychosocial rehabilitation services and a worker at Urban with a bachelor's degree in education pursuing a graduate degree in counseling.

At times, managers described how the labor market restricted whom they could hire. One manager at Suburban recounted trying to hire clinically trained staff in the past but falling short: "There was a period when, God, we couldn't hire people if we tried. It was just the job market. So I had someone who had a degree in English" (interview). At Urban, a manager explained how it was more difficult to find male and minority workers, given the dominance of White women in the field. "You pretty much can always find a White girl for a social service position," she said (interview). Steve, a male worker at Urban, tied this to the demographics of students in educational programs providing clinical training: "If you go to, you know, the grad school that I went to, the ratio of men to women was maybe one to fifteen, one to twenty. I think that matching demographics [between clients and workers] will always be a difficult prospect for any organization" (interview).

Those in charge of hiring described having to choose between the empowerment logic and the clinical-professional logic in deciding who was the best fit for a job. This is illustrated well by the considerations of staff in hiring for a few positions in the day program at Urban. The first position had been vacated by a prosumer and involved organizing the preparation of the day program's free lunch. It was a part-time position. When hiring to fill the position, staff members discussed the qualities desirable in a worker: One was someone who was a prosumer. Another was someone with some background in nutrition. The clients were "big meat eaters." Steve said the previous worker "showed compassion and connected with [clients] by serving lots of meat and very few vegetables" (field notes). However, staff and some clients thought meals should be healthier, and having someone experienced in nutrition would help move in that direction. When the hire was made, the worker was a prosumer without any professional background in nutrition or food preparation.

Evaluating candidates for the other two positions, Jessica initially discussed weighing the relative value of "education" versus "experience." One of the top candidates was a young White woman with an advanced degree; the other was a middle-aged Black woman without a degree but with years of experience working in another program within the organization. Both had applied for a "senior mental health worker" position, which was the first to be filled. However, Jessica kept in mind that a lower-ranking "mental health worker" position was also open. She ultimately decided to hire the White woman for the higher-ranking position and the African American woman for the lower-ranking position. Talking to me in an interview between the two hires, having just spoken in the interview of the importance of a diverse staff, Jessica made it clear that the racial background of the African American candidate was a factor in her hire. "Taking different things into consideration and things that were brought to the table in terms of who's going to fill the next position [the lower-ranking position], I believe that it will be an African American person" (interview). Jessica expressed consciously considering racial background, clinical credentials, and experience in hiring for these positions.

I could not verify the claims these workers made regarding the pool of applicants for positions. I did not collect data on applications for positions versus hires at either Urban or Suburban. There is some evidence that what employers say about hiring practices differs from what they actually do (Pager and Quillian 2005). National statistics may provide some insight; although statistics regarding the proportion of prosumers in behavioral health services are not readily available, demographic information regarding the mental health services field nationally is more easily accessible. Table 6.1 depicts the actual racial and gender variation in educational credentials in the fields commonly found in mental health services in the United States. The table shows the percentages of degrees and certificates completed at all levels in the 2006–2007 academic year. Although women and Whites made up the majority of completions in all fields, women's majority was dramatically larger in the fields related to mental health services: women made up nearly 60 percent of all degree and certificate completions, but made up 88 percent of social work completions and 75 percent of completions in mental and social services and allied professions.

Table 6.1. Degree Completions for Race and Gender in Mental Health Care Fields

Year: 2006–2007	Black	White	Men	Women
All degrees/certificates	11%	63%	41%	59%
Psychology	11%	66%	22%	78%
Social work	19%	60%	12%	88%
Human development/family studies and related services	18%	53%	6%	94%
Human services, general	26%	47%	18%	82%
Mental/social health services and allied professions	21%	60%	24%	76%
Rehabilitation/therapeutic professions	7%	73%	21%	79%

Source: Integrated Postsecondary Education Data System, National Center for Education Statistics.

African Americans' completions in these fields were also disproportionately larger, though they remained in the numerical minority. In the social work field, African Americans were 19 percent of completions and made up 21 percent in the mental and social health services and allied professions programs. Whites, on the other hand, who completed 66 percent of all degrees and certificate programs, remained near this proportion or dropped in fields related to mental health services, with the exception of rehabilitation and therapeutic professional programs. In no program did African Americans approach half of completions; Whites and women were the majority in all.

When we move from education to workers actually in the field, the pattern persists. Table 6.2 shows national statistics in the mental health care field. Though Blacks are disproportionately more likely to work in the occupations relating to mental health services than Whites, when it comes to management positions in social and community services, they are much less represented. Also visible here is the distinct gender imbalance, with women overrepresented in all professions related to mental health services yet still a minority in the overall labor force. This divergence based on race, age, personal experience, and rank led to distinct ways of relating to clients, and at times to tension among clients and different groups of workers.

I collected information on the makeup of workers at Urban and Suburban. There were, roughly speaking, two major groups of workers in both sites. The major dividing point was educational and clinical credentials, with one group

Table 6.2. Labor Force Participation for Race and Gender in Mental Health Care Fields

Year: 2008	Black	White	Men	Women
Total labor force	11%	82%	53%	47%
Social/community service managers	10%	84%	32%	68%
Miscellaneous community and social service specialists	21%	73%	39%	61%
Social workers	25%	71%	21%	79%
Counselors	20%	73%	32%	68%
Nursing, psychiatric, and home health aids	35%	58%	11%	89%

Source: Unpublished table, Bureau of Labor Statistics.

having many and the other generally lacking them. However, this characteristic correlated with others, and so the groups tended to differ in other ways. Clinically credentialed staff tended to be younger and were often hired fresh out of school (whether graduate or undergraduate). Workers without credentials, on the other hand, were more likely to have lived other lives before entering the behavioral health services field. Some had had completely different careers, ranging from fashion modeling to finance to janitorial. Both organizations' workers without clinical credentials were more likely to be racial ethnic minorities—especially African American—and to be prosumers. These workers without clinical credentials tended to hold lower positions in the organizations. In some ways, it should not be a surprise that those with more clinical credentials tended to hold positions with more power and prestige at both Suburban and Urban. Within the mental health field, state Medicaid regulations enforced the hierarchy through their clinical requirements on who could hold certain positions.

Institutional Logics, Worker Background, and Client Relations

In her analysis of post-reform welfare bureaucracies, Celeste Watkins-Hayes (2009) finds that, for Black and Latino welfare caseworkers, racial and ethnic background issues are an unavoidable part of their job. These workers engage in what Watkins-Hayes refers to as "racialized professionalism," deciding whether and how to use their own race (and their relatively privileged positions) to connect with their race-mate clients, helping them to make sense of and navigate the welfare system. She also finds that personal experience with poverty and with being clients in the welfare system also play a role in worker's dealings with clients. Steven Maynard-Moody and Michael Musheno (2003) describe how numerous identity categories that workers and clients occupy—not only race, but also gender, age, disability status, and professional background—affect interactions between different groups of workers and between workers and clients. Managers in the mental health field—calling on the empowerment logic—understand this and see it as an asset, using race, gender, personal experience with mental illness or addiction, and other background characteristics as criteria in hiring workers. However, the resulting division among staff led to two distinct ways of relating to clients, which embodied the logics that underlay hiring.

Clinically trained staff members were more likely to deal with clients using the clinical-professional logic, building relationships with strict boundaries and a clinical, abstract analysis of clients' situations. Staff without clinical training, on the other hand, tended to relate to clients on a more personal level, operating on the peer support principle of the empowerment logic. They emphasized their own experience with the issues clients faced and built relationships based on that shared background. These different approaches constituted different professional personas that members of the different groups adopted in interacting with clients.

Worker Personas

Because of their clinical training and their relative social distance from clients—in terms of race, class, age, and, often, socioeconomic status—clinically trained workers were generally much more conscious of and focused on the *clinical persona* they adopted in their relationships with clients. Most of these workers consciously interacted with clients in ways different from how they interacted with others. A major component of this was maintaining boundaries between themselves and clients. These staff attempted to maintain asymmetrical relationships with clients, sharing much less of their own lives with clients than clients shared with them (Estroff 1981)—being personable, but not personal.[2] The clinical persona aimed for "affective neutrality" (Parsons 1951)—to be objective, not emotional.

This dynamic was captured well by Katie, a young White intern at Urban. Katie came from a privileged background and recognized the distance between her own life experience and that of clients. She detailed actively trying to manage how she presented herself to clients.

I mean clients tell me in groups, like, "What do you know about crack addiction?" or like "You're my daughter's age," you know? And they're absolutely right. I was worried—conscious about acting too professionally because it is also a friendly environment. . . . And so, I was like, "Well, how do I act like a professional friend?" or like somebody who is friendly but professional at the same time? . . . And I have worried sometimes that I have been either too intimate towards participants [or] that I am being too distant. Sometimes I worry that I have talked kind of condescend- ingly towards participants. . . . [My supervisor] told me that I need to think about my affect [in dealing with clients]. I said, "Well, what could I change in me?" He said, "You are very happy. It is like you are always smiling." . . . Then I thought—and I got to think, you know, "Why am I so happy . . . ?" And then think about, "Am I falsely happy? Am I not falsely happy? Should I continue to act the way that I am because that is me, or, you know, is it not professional enough?" (interview)

It is as revealing that her internship supervisor addressed the issue with her as it is that Katie consciously focused on how she presented herself to clients; it is an important focus of the clinical-professional logic. "Professional boundar- ies" are erected and carefully maintained between service professionals and the clients they serve. Doing so, the clinical logic dictates, keeps the focus on how best to meet clients' clinical needs and helps avoid exploitation and manipula- tion in the relationship. The clinical supervision of boundaries and interaction with clients was also evidenced by Glenda. She described working with a staff member—one who interacted with clients in a "parental" and "punitive" man- ner—to help the staff member develop a more clinically informed demeanor.

There was situation where [a client who hallucinates frequently was standing] right outside an office door. I was there and the staff member responded in a pretty rude manner: "What are you doing?" . . . I said, "That was rude. That was pretty rude." And the staff member said, "Well, they were just standing out there." I said, "That—you know that's an individual who hallucinates. Do you think they really were tuned in to what we were saying? And wouldn't you want to shape their behavior? How does [responding in that way] teach them to do anything different? Don't you want to say, 'You may need something but what you need to do is knock on the door, and say, "I would like to talk to you," and then we can then say, "In five minutes, I'll come and get you."'" Wouldn't that be better?" And so this individual does see that, and sees more and more of that, but it's been a lot of work—working away from the punitive . . . to really a therapeutic model of shaping and modeling. (interview)

Instead of correcting clients in the familiar way, as a worker might speak to his or her own child, Glenda suggests the staff member adopt a careful clinical persona, one informed by the clinical logic.

For staff members with clinical training, workers' disclosure of their personal information or experiences to clients was seen as risky and was in many circumstances discouraged. Fremont, a White manager at Urban, held advanced clinical credentials but also had dealt with mental illness and substance abuse in his past. He nevertheless adopted the clinical persona when talking about worker self-disclosure with clients. He said that although his own experiences might be evident to clients indirectly, he had not disclosed his past outright. In general he thought it was a bad idea, and his explanation was a common one among staff with clinical credentials.

> I think, you know, the general rule is . . . if and when you disclose anything, it has to be one hundred percent for the benefit of the client. . . . It cannot be about yourselves, cannot be about you. If so, it's not appropriate. You never do it to build credibility, because a lot of times . . . [a staff member discloses something about his or her life, and] they get two opposing reactions from different clients and [even] from the same client. . . . [On the positive side, a client might say,] "He's been there. He knows what I've gone through." So they have a bond and a better, you know—not better—but a therapeutic alliance based on that. But when they're disagreeing, that same participant will say, "Who the hell is he to tell me what to do?"—even if they're not telling him what to do. "He's just dope fiend like me," you know. "He's just a drunk," you know. "He's doing this for that reason." "Oh he's relapsed." . . . I've heard all of those things . . . [Disclosing to clients] doesn't build credibility . . . I think a lot of times that the benefits are really outweighed by the pitfalls and the drawbacks of it . . . The better we are at what we do the less necessity there is to self-disclose. At the same time . . . there are ways that it works its way in. (interview)

To Fremont and many other clinically oriented workers—especially those not possessing personal characteristics tying them to clients—self-disclosure was a fallback tool used by those without sufficient skills to interact with clients in the most clinically effective ways. Even though he saw some value in connecting with clients based on shared background, Fremont felt that such connections were risky and that effective clinical skills obviated the need to call on those characteristics in working with clients.

In their classic study of a psychiatric hospital, Anselm Strauss et al. (1963) note that psychiatric aides, who lacked the professional training that nurses and psychiatrists possessed but who interacted with patients more frequently and more openly than professionals, had distinct ways of interacting with patients. They also had unique criteria for judging client progress, guided by "common-sense maxims" rather than by technical-clinical knowledge. Workers with little formal clinical training are also common in contemporary community care (Dill 2001). Anne Scott (2012) argues that peer support workers in mental health services engage in what she calls "authenticity work." These staff members engage in distinct forms of emotional labor, managing weaker boundaries with clients than other professionals. They incorporate into their work concerns with mutuality, honesty, and sharing with clients. The sharing she refers to is regarding workers' own history with mental distress.

For workers at Urban and Suburban without clinical credentials, shared experiences with clients could involve not only homelessness, drugs, prison, or mental illness, but also racial/ethnic background, gender, or age. These workers used personal experiences and characteristics not as a fallback but as a primary basis of interaction. They presented an *authentic persona* in their interactions with clients. They were much less concerned with erecting boundaries between their personal lives and clients. What they brought to the interaction was more wisdom than clinical insight. Workers from this group felt that this mode of interaction gave them legitimacy in the eyes of clients, which clinically trained workers lacked. Lorena, a White prosumer at Urban, said sometimes she shared with clients that she takes medication when they are struggling with taking theirs:

I think that when the participants are struggling with taking medication I'll tell them that I take medication and I'll say it makes me feel better, you know. I don't go into depth, but I'll kind of run over [it]. . . . Then I'll tell them about my homelessness, but I don't disclose it to everybody. . . . But I want them to know that I've been where they've been, you know, and it is helpful to them. So when I feel that it would be of aid to them, I'll say, "Oh," you know, "I was homeless too, and I was walking around these streets," or if they're struggling with being at the shelter, I'll say, "Yeah, I know what you mean, I was there, too." . . . I think it's very helpful to them. (interview)

Though she was not completely open with everyone about her background, Lorena did disclose her shared experience with some of the issues clients dealt with. Some clients responded well to this type of disclosure. For instance, Shauntee, a Black client at Urban, described how a White outreach worker telling her he took medication made her feel more comfortable seeking help for her issues: "At first I was like leery because I didn't really know them. . . . And what really made me go ahead to sign up [was] because Stefan told me that he take[s] medication. So, when he said that, then that made me go ahead and sign up. He was being honest" (interview). Trust is a major factor in worker-client relations (Hasenfeld 2010a), and a worker adopting the authentic persona—being honest about their own background when that background was shared with clients—could help build that trusting relationship.

There were other points of connection between workers and clients in the authentic persona. Age and race were also significant. Barry, a middle-aged Black worker at Suburban without a college degree or any clinical credentials (other than years of experience working in the field), talked about how his race, gender, and age allowed him to make connections with and help some clients in ways other workers were not able to do.

> I guess I kind of bring a "macho man" kind of persona . . . I probably relate to the guys a little differently than most of the other guys [that work here], and so I think in that sense that's actually a good thing. I—I know that I made some good connections. . . . My relationship with Phillip. Um, you know—one, he's Black, I'm Black, and I think that, for him, has been a really good thing. And I could see, you know, to a certain extent it's been helpful, for me, in terms of being able to talk to him. . . . There's some times I can help him, kind of deal with the situation in a way that he doesn't necessarily feel that [his worker, a young White woman] can. . . . It's just, you know, generationally he and I are, you know, we're just about the same age. I kind of understand what he's saying and that's—we can speak on it. And then I could kind of—I can challenge him in a way that [his worker], you know, just can't do.

For Barry, the shared background characteristics were not simply a means of "breaking the ice," though they definitely served that purpose. His background was also a tool he used to "challenge" Phillip regarding issues Phillip was dealing with, a means to do mental health work. Staff who shared clients' background were able to use their own experiences as role models for clients, saying they had gone through what clients had gone through and therefore knew the difficulties firsthand (Watkins-Hayes 2009). Their challenges to clients were based not on clinical theories but instead on workers' own triumphs and tribulations. From this viewpoint, client successes and failures had implications for the broader groups (race, gender, mental health consumer) to which they and the workers belonged.

Race was particularly powerful among the various characteristics that could influence hiring under the empowerment logic and thus underlay interaction in the authentic persona. Because of its visibility and resonance in everyday life, Black workers and clients gave race special significance. Further, because of its correlation with other characteristics possessed by workers hired under the empowerment logic—personal experience with clinical issues, age, and socioeconomic status, for example—minority workers and clients at times used race as a proxy for groups of these characteristics when discussing interaction based on the authentic persona.

Even when Black workers possessed or were pursuing clinical credentials, they nevertheless were more likely to adopt the authentic persona than were their White counterparts. Henry, an African American mental health worker at Suburban, had an associate's degree in nursing. Although his specialization in nursing was not mental health, the credential could bring him some educational credibility. It could not, however, lead to him being promoted above mental health professional (MHP) status, one step above RSA. He also had a history of drug dealing, drug abuse, and prison. Most of the clients at Urban were Black, and they sometimes had trouble building relationships with White staff members, according to Henry. He felt that his background aided him in building relationships and working with clients at Urban, which he claimed he could do as well as or better than his more clinically trained colleagues.

> Most of the staff—I'd say 99 percent of them don't have—don't have racial problems with reaching clients. *Clients* have problems with having faith in White-Caucasian people because a lot of the [service providers who disappointed them in the past were White]. . . . You know a lot of my colleagues have, you know, their master's and . . . their [clinical] license. And though we may be in the same job, they make more money. And that's cool—they earn it. Okay, but the point is I can give the same effect or, or they might admire how, how a client responds to me, you know. . . . If I'm gone for a couple of weeks, clients will really get, you know, antsy. "Where is Henry?" you know. It's a piece that allows them to feel like, because I've been there that—that "I'm going to get a fair shake because he's around." They're gonna get a fair shake anyway,

but for them, "I'm going to get a fair shake because that guy's around."
(interview)

Though he had fewer clinical credentials than some other workers, Henry did
have a college degree. Nevertheless, he felt that some of the most useful things
he brought to his relationships with clients were his personal background and
experiences. Though he saw his colleagues as very skilled, he felt his experiences endowed him with a different kind of skill, albeit one that was less
rewarded with pay and rank.

One reason why workers who had both clinical training and shared background with clients might opt for the authentic persona rather than the clinical
persona in interacting with clients was that professional clinical training itself
might clash with the workers' own background (Costello 2005; Karp 1986).
Sociologists since W.E.B. Du Bois (1904) have pointed out that racial/ethnic
minorities have had to develop a "double consciousness" in order to "straddle
boundaries" (Carter 2006) between their home cultures and those of the White-
dominated society. Dealing specifically with professional training of lawyers
and social workers, Carrie Yang Costello (2005) describes how students from
minority and low socioeconomic status backgrounds experience "identity dissonance" in the process of reconciling their former identity with that developed
socializing into the culture of professional school, revealing a White, middle-
class bias to the professional training. This dissonance could lead to students
having problems in personal relationships with friends and family more accustomed to the former identity. Some dealt with this by splitting their identities,
acting distinctly differently depending on with whom they interacted—being
professional in the professional setting and more familiar with friends and family. This implies that interaction with clients based on shared background may
not be easy to pull off seamlessly.

When a worker possessing both personal experience and professional
training interacts with clients, an integrated identity may not be what is presented, and workers may choose the authentic persona to the exclusion of the
professional persona. This tension was evident in the comments of one Black
client recounting his interaction with a Black worker with some clinical training whom he accused of "picking at" him. He said the worker replied to his
complaints with the following response: "What you want me to be? You want
me to be White? Be like them? Sell myself out?" For this worker, interactions
with the client were characterized by shared familiar racial interaction patterns,
and the client's questioning of those interactions—perhaps calling for more
"clinical" interactions—were tantamount to asking the worker to "be White."

The dissonance between professional training and workers' backgrounds could prevent integration into a unified identity, leading them to opt for interaction based on shared background rather than clinical training.

Social Control and Labeling

In chapter 3, I discussed how, regardless of the official labels applied to clients for the purposes of bureaucracy and resource channeling, workers also applied informal labels regarding client mental illness. These labels, when combined with informal labels regarding client disruptiveness, led to different types of responses to clients. When clients were informally labeled *symptomatic*, staff responded to disruptions with *medicalizing responses.* Workers absolved these clients of moral judgment and gave them much more leeway in violating organizational rules and routines. On the other hand, if clients were not labeled symptomatic, then staff responded to them with *moralizing responses*, thus holding them accountable for rule violations. Clinically trained staff and staff hired based on the empowerment logic not only tended to be hired on different bases and have different patterns of interacting with clients, but also had different patterns of informally labeling clients. Staff without clinical training were less likely to view clients as symptomatic than clinically trained workers and were more likely to respond to rule violations with moralizing responses.

This could be seen at Suburban in the tension between the workshop portion of the program and the rest of the day program. The workshop put clients to work in light assembly or in packing boxes for outside customers who contracted with Suburban. The number of clients working there and the volume of work had been substantial in the past but had dropped markedly in the years leading up to my time there. The provider received a waiver from the state so clients could be paid piece rate, meaning clients were paid a percentage of minimum wage based on how fast they worked—few were paid at or above minimum wage. Though there was a schedule, it was not strictly enforced, and some clients came and went without much regard to the schedule. This presented problems in achieving efficient management.

The White manager in charge of the workshop, Leo, had a bachelor's degree in the arts but did not have clinical training, though he had worked with the workshop for many years. Although he was officially in a supervisory position according to state regulation, he was only an MHP, which limited his ability to supervise others clinically. The approach he took to the workshop was to treat it as much like external employment as possible, because he had real orders coming in that he needed to fill and customers he must answer to. He attempted therefore to hold clients who participated in the workshop to high expectations. This was illustrated in his description of an interaction with a client who habitually did not show up as scheduled and did not call him to let him know she was not coming. "I tried to put some weight on. 'This is ridiculous. I'm going to be suspending you. If this was a real job, I'd be firing you. You've got to at least call me up'" (interview). He argued broadly for clients not to be allowed to deviate from their schedule and not to be allowed to come and go from the workshop unscheduled (for example, when they were bored or did not have other things to do), but was overruled by the overall program director (field notes). Instead of viewing clients through the clinical lens and calling for flexibility, as did the program director, Leo more frequently moralized clients, evaluating them by what would happen in the "real world" and holding them to a higher standard.

Because of the high correlation between race and clinical training, worker discussion of differences in social control often revolved around race. Black staff members at both organizations talked about how they interacted with clients differently than White staff members did. They reported how White staff members were more likely to allow clients to be disrespectful and were less likely to correct clients. For example, Nina, a Black woman worker at Urban, said that, in her view,

I think that the White workers tend to be more easygoing—easy, period. . . . Some, not all—some. They believe the little games and the manip[ulation]—and I'm just sitting here [shakes head]. Some of the Black workers [do it] too, now don't get me wrong. But the majority is the White workers. They always want to talk real nice and soft. That's not needed some—that's not needed all the time. Sometimes you have to be like, "Look, you need to cut this shit out. Stop it, because you know what you're doing." Like, for instance, [a Black female client]: she be in the kitchen just stirring it up, and you just have to tell her—and be firm. There are a lot of times that I don't think people be firm and follow through with what they say. Like, "I'm gonna have to ask you to leave." You keep having that conversation: "Look it's time for you to go," you know. "You been warned several times. It's time for you to go. If you do not leave, I'm calling the police," and stick to that and call the police. See, you've got the follow through and just be firm. Some Black workers are like that, too. But my approach is—they're always calling me mean, but I'm not being mean. (interview)

Nina appeared to informally label the clients she discusses as bad; she argues that they "know what [they're] doing," implying an ability to control their disruptive behaviors. She described herself and other Black workers as calling out clients more frequently than White staff members did.

Workers with clinical credentials, calling on their body of expert knowledge, appeared more likely to view client disruptions as symptoms of illness, whereas those without that training emphasized calling on life experience outside of the confines of the organization. If the workers were prosumers, this experience could be their own firsthand dealings with the issues facing clients. If they were not, their basis of judgment could be how these disruptions would be dealt with by the average person outside the facility's setting. For example, at Suburban, Barry talked about his reaction to a young White male client who had frequent aggressive outbursts: "Brother, you can do that here, because no one's going to do anything to you. You do that in the real world to the wrong person, you're gonna have some problems" (field notes). If the worker without clinical credentials had witnessed the client act in a controlled, competent manner in the past or in a different setting, that could be used as evidence that the client was capable and should be judged as such. Bobby, a Black prosumer worker at Urban, illustrated this in his discussion of a client that "bullies" some staff: "He knows honestly what he's doing because he's been, in the past, in one of the treatment centers that I've worked in. And his whole attitude was different there" (interview). Assuming the client was in control of his behavior, Bobby took the client aside and made a point to correct him, something that Bobby said the more clinically trained (White) workers were not willing to do. Clinically trained workers were less likely to expect such consistency in client behavior. They instead might refer to such changes in behavior as "decompensation" or the "cyclical" nature of a client's mental illness, as I witnessed in staff meetings (field notes), and react accordingly.

Logics, Staffing, and Hierarchy

Resolving the institutional fragmentation between the empowerment and clinical-professional logics in hiring led to two groups of workers with different ways of interacting with clients. These two groups were not simply different, however. They were also given different levels of power and prestige within the organization. Although the importance of including peer support in the organization was acknowledged, both regulative and normative institutionalization rendered it secondary and subordinate to the clinical-professional logic.

State regulations required clinical credentials for workers to hold certain classifications in providing Medicaid-reimbursable services. Those without clinical credentials were generally hired in as either RSAs, the lowest rank, or as MHPs, the next step up. RSAs required no credentials or experience, whereas MHPs needed to have either a bachelor's degree or experience working in the field. Any higher ranks, such as QMHP (Qualified Mental Health Professional) or LPHA, required advanced or specialized degrees or clinical licensure. So, the major form of advancement available for those without clinical credentials was to work in the field and move up to MHP. If a new hire had already worked in the field and thus started as an MHP, further advancement was not possible without further education or certification. For much of my time at Urban, the position of clinical manager of the case management teams was vacant. Vinnie, an Asian worker and an MHP, was promoted to fill the position for a time. However, he lost the position when it became clear that someone serving in that capacity had to be at least a QMHP. Vinnie had only a bachelor's degree and was not licensed. He had no interest in obtaining an advanced degree and so was demoted (field notes). The person eventually hired for the position had both an advanced degree and licensure.

In addition to lacking credentials to move beyond RSA or MHP positions, prosumers had other restrictions on their ability to advance within the organizations. Many worked part time for a couple of reasons. First, the positions for which they were hired were often designated as part-time positions, so they had little choice in the matter even if they wanted to increase their hours. However, another reason they often worked part time was by their own choice. Full-time work was seen as simply too stressful for many prosumers dealing with severe mental illness. Further, if they were receiving Social Security work disability benefits, these staff members were limited in the amount of money they could make in a given year without losing their benefits. Just as clients feared losing this secure source of income, prosumers were anxious about it as well. Full-time work would put them over that limit quickly. Even with part-time work, one prosumer at Urban took extended absences so as to not exceed her income limit (field notes).

What this meant for daily mental health work is that those most likely to be in charge of the organization came from a clinically trained background. Their knowledge and their means of interacting were officially sanctioned and were given more power and prestige. They supervised workers without clinical training and so were in positions to decide how and when the less-clinically informed ways of dealing with clients were "appropriate" and advisable. Clinically trained workers saw problems with prosumers working without close clinical supervision. For instance, a manager at Suburban revealed this in discussing peer programs staffed by prosumers without significant clinical training: "My great fear is that they probably occasionally do some really whopper errors and that has to get fixed up and/or people are hurt again, you know?" (interview). Further, the ways of interacting with clients that workers without clinical training used at times were seen as problematic by clinically trained workers, who were in a position to enforce their viewpoints. Monique was a Black female worker at Suburban with a bachelor's degree in education (not a clinical field) who was pursuing graduate work in the mental health field. She admitted that she talked to clients in a "parental" manner and that she had been told by her White supervisor her that manner of interaction was "rude" and not clinically appropriate:

> [My supervisor] tells me I need to work on—how I speak [to clients] . . .
> I am just very direct. I am not mean. I am just direct. I said—or I think
> sometimes [whispers], "Do you think I need to talk like this, [supervisor's name]? Is that what you think?" [Back to normal volume] No, [my
> supervisor] said I need to watch out, "Even the tone." . . . because I have
> got a "mommy tone." (interview)

With the reference to the possibility she might be viewed as "mean," we can see the resemblance between Monique's comments and those of Nina above. This type of clinical oversight of the authentic persona was common at both organizations. I even heard reports (though I did not observe this myself) that workers had resigned and had been fired over related issues at Urban.

The gist of the clinically trained staff's perspective on workers without clinical training—who were more likely to share client characteristics—was that they were good to have around, but that they had more issues in their work that needed to be "managed" or "supported" with close monitoring by people with clinical credentials. Steve, a clinically trained worker from Urban, expressed this position well.

> I think that there needs to be more support. I think that the agency needs
> to build support systems around [prosumers]. And I think that [Urban]
> actually—they could actually use some improvement in the area.
> Because I think as—as much as line staff across the board need support, I think that prosumers have, in some instances, more challenges
> and more obstacles. They may not have, you know, bachelor's, they may
> not have master's degree, may not have been exposed to ethics, rules,

expectations, you know, counseling styles, approaches, etc. And I think ongoing training and, you know, close supervision is very good. You know, I think the prosumers, you know, have a higher susceptibility of falling into, closely, to relationships with the participants. They can be vulnerable to participants. (interview)

This vulnerability included an increased likelihood of disclosure of personal information, which, like Fremont, Steve thought was risky.

Although, as Strauss et al. (1963) argue, organizational reality is a negotiation in which no group is completely without power, in these mental health care organizations those with clinical credentials, who had more organizational power than those without them, could negotiate much more successfully.

Discussion and Conclusion

The distribution of clinical credentials at Urban and Suburban was correlated with other worker characteristics, such as race, age, and gender. Prospective White workers—especially White women—were more likely to obtain clinically related degrees, certificates, and licenses. They were also more likely to be hired—based on the clinical logic—for higher-ranking positions (or promoted into those positions) within the organization. On the other hand, the organizations more frequently hired non-credentialed workers—who were more often Black, older, and male—using the empowerment logic, seeing value in their backgrounds and personal experiences that could facilitate relationships with clients. Thus, this bifurcated workforce had two distinct ways of interacting with clients, reflecting the different institutional logics used to hire them. Workers without clinical credentials saw their clinically trained coworkers as more likely not to hold clients accountable for disruptive behavior. Uncredentialed workers, calling on concrete evidence of client capability, more commonly constructed labels of clients as not symptomatic and approached them with moralizing responses. Institutional fragmentation in the process of hiring was manifested in a fragmented work force.

Although some of the core values of the empowerment logic were recognized—even touted—by workers, administrators, clinicians, and policymakers, their implementation in staffing by workers occupying the highest levels within organizations was limited, both by policies governing the organizations and by workers' own values. State policies pushed mental health organizations they fund toward the clinical logic and away from the empowerment logic in hiring for upper-level positions. Despite this, there is evidence that such workers can actually be effective in working with clients in ways that clinically trained workers cannot—even more effective in defusing client resistance when this resistance is itself based in race, class, or gender (Gengler 2012).

This leads to the question of exactly how much these organizations and the state in which they were located truly valued peer support in their staff. It is clear that having staff members who shared client background brought legitimacy to the providers. Having workers who had "been there" gave the organizations ways to connect to clients who otherwise would have avoided them or engaged in services much less quickly or fully. Further, with their more frank, familiar, and somewhat stricter interaction with clients, workers sharing client background were willing and able to regulate clients more than other workers. However, because of the inverse correlation between sharing client background and possessing clinical credentials, these workers were limited in advancement potential. Government regulations institutionalized a preference for clinical educational credentials. Within the structure of Medicaid reimbursement, there was only so much value that could be formally given to a peer background. Though it may help them obtain a lower level job at Urban or Suburban, without further educational attainment these workers were stuck at the bottom of the organizational hierarchy.

The processes I analyze within this chapter were present at both Urban and Suburban, but because of the distinct demographics of staff and clients at the two organizations, there were differences in how the processes played out. At Suburban, where a small fraction of both clients and workers were Black, close bonds based on racial background affected relatively few staff. Further, problems with substance abuse, prison, and homelessness were much less common among both staff and clients there. The personal experiences that uncredentialed staff members called upon in bonding with clients at Suburban were thus more likely to be rooted in other demographic characteristics (gender, age) and in experience with mental illness. Nevertheless, because of the differences in clinical credentials, there was a difference in how credentialed and noncredentialed staff members there interacted with clients, as noted above.

At Urban, most of the clients were Black, and so Black workers shared most clients' racial background. Further, most of the Black staff members at Urban were prosumers, so they shared not only racial/ethnic background and age with clients, but also the struggle with mental illness, substance abuse, homelessness, or prison. So not only were shared backgrounds between Black staff members and clients at Urban more common, they were also based on a wider range of experiences. Though the present data do not allow a full analysis of this issue, it seems logical that frustrations at Urban regarding racial hierarchy, which I did not detect at Suburban, could be grounded in thoughts that the Black workers at Urban considered themselves experts in clinical issues confronting clients because, although they might not have the formal training other workers had, they had dealt with the issues personally. From this viewpoint, they could be seen in some sense as being as qualified as those with formal training who themselves lack that personal experience.

There is hope for those advocating for more formal recognition and advancement of peer support in public mental health care. Organizations do exist in which peer support workers make up the majority of—if not all—employees (Clay et al. 2005; McLean 2000). However, as stated earlier, these tend to be funded by grants and not with more-stable Medicaid funding. Even within organizations with a mix of peer and non-peer employees, formal recognition of the value of sharing client background is growing. For instance, in Massachusetts, entry-level employees in publicly contracted mental health care are paid a higher salary if they have a background as a mental health consumer than are those without that background.[3] These instances, although currently rare and precarious, are becoming more common. Hope exists for those wanting change in the clinical logic as well, with some challenging the logic's emphasis on affective neutrality and the enforcement of strict boundaries between clients and workers (for example, Comstock et al. 2008). However, to the degree that the current clinical logic is institutionalized in mental health regulation as the primary basis of judging worker qualifications, the empowerment logic will always be subordinate. In this context, workers wanting to bring shared background with clients to the higher levels of organizational hierarchy in publicly funded mental health care will only be able to do so by adding clinical credentials to their resumes.

Chapter 7

Conclusion

A patient or worker entrenched in the mental health system of the early twentieth century would be astounded by what they would find in today's system. Instead of a field dominated by state hospitals, they would find hospitals an increasingly small component of the mental health care sector. Instead, with the ascent of the community logic, community care is now the preferred site of services. As a result, a progressively dizzying array of community organizations—not only behavioral, but also housing, public welfare, and other providers—offer services that were once centralized in the hospital setting. The logics guiding the system have also changed—and proliferated. Instead of the formerly dominant clinical-professional logic holding sway over the field, other logics exist alongside it, affecting how care is delivered. The civil rights and consumer movements led to the formation of the empowerment logic in the late 1960s. Client voices are now considered a legitimate consideration in care. Further, the logic of bureaucratic accountability acts as a constant source of checks on professional practice, which holds cost-containment and tracking outcomes as more important than protecting professional prerogative.

These logics continue to coexist, and they do not always agree on the recommended course of action. Should workers push clients to be more independent because it would lead to greater community integration, or should they allow clients to choose to be dependent on the organization because that is what the clients say they want? Instances of institutional fragmentation such as this are countless in contemporary care for people with severe mental illness.

How these types of conflicts are resolved is highly influenced by how the logics involved are institutionalized. The empowerment logic was well institutionalized normatively; in the mental health sector and in organizational rhetoric, client self-determination, peer support, and helping clients remove barriers to success all received widespread endorsement. I found relatively few regulatory imperatives tied to the logic, however. Those that did exist were not tied to funding or were easy for workers to circumvent when they felt it appropriate. This was consequential when workers experienced institutional fragmentation involving the empowerment logic, because the other logics involved—the logic of bureaucratic accountability and the community logic—were much more firmly institutionalized in regulation. This translated into more severe consequences for the provider if they opted for the empowerment logic over the other—often a loss of funding. Deciding against the empowerment logic rarely had the same consequences. Thus, the empowerment logic often lost out.

At times worker responses were not a simple either-or decision. Staff found workarounds or other adaptations to meet the seemingly contradictory requirements of more than one logic. For instance, providers would apply a less-than-optimal official diagnosis despite informational problems—satisfying the bureaucratic logic—while informally continuing to adjust their actual labels of clients over time when new information arose—respecting the clinical logic. Similarly, workers' use of "practical empowerment" allowed them to give clients some choice but, at the same time, help them make the choices staff preferred, whatever the reason. This reason could be the staff's clinical judgment, but it could also be more a practical reason, such as staff needing to make up billable hours.

Though institutional fragmentation was a central component of the dynamics within both organizations, it was not the only factor influencing day-to-day life there. Inequality, among both clients and staff, was also important. The relative poverty of the clients at Urban framed much of what happened there. Those clients who had developed skills to survive in the situation of deprivation were able to use those skills to direct the organization's resources toward themselves. Further, the increasing inequality in the gentrifying neighborhood in which Urban was located affected the ability of clients to integrate into the community. Among staff at both organizations, those workers who were more likely to be disadvantaged in the outside world—racial/ethnic minority workers, those with mental illness and substance abuse histories, and those with less education or training—also tended to be at the bottom of the organizational hierarchy, even though their experience and method of working with clients were valued.

Theoretical Contributions

Patterned ways of acting and thinking—ways that may or may not be officially endorsed—become established, maintained, and changed in organizations. Cultural scripts or "rational myths" can be adopted by organizations for reasons other than efficiency or effectiveness (DiMaggio and Powell 1983; Meyer and Rowan 1977). The legitimacy and resources brought by such "ceremonial" adoption is more important than the intended purpose of the adopted elements. This leads to a decoupling of organizational structure and day-to-day practice—for instance, graduation ceremonies and the hiring of licensed teachers can be disconnected from what actually goes on in the classroom (Meyer and Rowan 1978). We saw this sort of decoupling in the differing functions of official and informal labels in the organizations. The requirement of the bureaucratic logic that resource provision be legitimized through "medical necessity" forced workers to apply diagnoses they might not really believe. In actual mundane practice, however, the clinical logic underlay informal labels that dictated how workers interacted with clients. Mental health and other human services fields are often referred to as highly institutionalized—versus technical—because the outcomes of services are difficult to measure (Meyer 1986; Scott and Meyer 1991). In such environments, myth, ceremony, and decoupling happen frequently.

Technology itself can be rooted in the logics dominating a field (Hasenfeld 2010b; Thornton, Ocasio, and Lounsbury 2012). In mental health care, the logic of bureaucratic accountability was not a major force in care for people with severe mental illness in all historical periods. In modern times, taking its cues from the rise of managed care in the broader health care field, and mirroring similar efforts in the education field (Hallett 2010), the mental health care sector began to focus attention on cost-containment, accountability, and measurement of outcomes (Scheid 2003; Scheid 2004; Schlesinger and Gray 1999). Such efforts led to changes in the ways services were delivered, even if the goal was not the improvement of those services (Scheid 2003).

Logics affect micro-level dynamics within organizations (Barley 2008; Hallett and Ventresca 2006; Thornton, Ocasio, and Lounsbury 2012). With numerous logics circulating in a field, any organizational setting can have several logics at play, competing for or divided in organizational influence. For instance, in her study of a transitional housing organization, Amy Binder (2007) found that distinct units within the same organization respond to institutional pressures in different ways. Further, dependence on federal funds affected units differently. In one department with a great degree of professionalization among staff, workers creatively balanced demands attached to funding with other professionally informed concerns in a process Binder refers to as *bricolage*. Another department that was similarly dependent on federal funds, but which lacked professionalized staff, was much more concerned with adherence to regulatory guidelines (see also Heimer 1999).

So, broad logics interact with meaning-making inside organizations. But not all logics become embedded—or institutionalized—into organizational life in the same way. Recall that W. Richard Scott emphasized that institutions (and their attendant logics)[1] rest on three "pillars"—normative, cognitive, and regulative. Which pillar logics are built upon matters, especially when logics conflict. The logic that is dominant can vary over time (Scott et al. 2000), and one factor affecting that dominance is how the different logics become embedded in organizational life. Regulative institutionalization is essential if the goal is to constrain behavior. Clear behavioral guidelines and strict enforcement ensure behavior even when values and cognitive schemas are lacking, or when they conflict. This is especially the case in fields where public funding and policy play major roles, such as care for people with severe mental illness and other human services fields.

Institutional change in the mental health care sector set the stage for battles for clinical autonomy with providers (Schlesinger and Gray 1999). With the spread of the tools such as utilization review and medical necessity, providers increasingly have to justify their decisions in order to receive the funds to continue providing care. The mental health sector has weaker professionalization and fewer clear outcomes to measure than the medical field, so the constraints on provider practice are even more pronounced there than in the medical sector (Scheid and Greenberg 2007; Schlesinger and Gray 1999).

The clinical-professional logic, the empowerment logic, the logic of bureaucratic accountability, and the community logic all bear on numerous aspects of frontline mental health care service delivery. The demands of the logics might be weighed and considered in the abstract—for example, the community logic and bureaucratic accountability (Bond 2004) or the empowerment logic and bureaucratic accountability (Anthony, Rogers, and Farkas 2003)—but reconciliation is not simply an abstract exercise. It is a practical problem, one confronting staff at every turn. As the field evolves, organizations and their workers must continually make decisions, weighing values and consequences of implementing one logic or another. The patterns that result reveal which logic is dominant. So, commodification (which I frame as part of the logic of bureaucratic accountability) may push out the professional logic, focusing on cost-containment to the exclusion of improving standards of care (Scheid 2003).

Workers are pulled in conflicting directions, sometimes at a loss for which way to go. How logics are institutionalized strongly shapes workers actions, but workers also develop adaptive routines and shortcuts, such as informal labeling and practical empowerment.

Implications for Policy and Practice

"The central problem for . . . policy is translation" (Bryson 2005). This statement is as true for mental health policy as it is for cultural policy. Focusing on "street-level" practice shows us realities we would never see by simply looking at rules and regulations as written (Lipsky 1980). In much the same way, looking at one institutional logic in a field obscures the very real competition between logics characterizing the evolution of fields over time. Though dominant logics may change, those that are displaced often persist (Scott et al. 2000).

A key issue for policy translation is how logics are embedded in a field. Though rules and procedures are formed at the organizational level, I have focused on how field-level institutionalization penetrates organizations, shaping both administration and street-level practice. Although professional norms, consumer advocacy, and academic research all play major roles at the field level in normative and cognitive institutionalization, much of the most powerful institutionalization—regulative—comes from government policymakers and accrediting organizations (which often work in tandem). These policymakers appear to have limited ability to control normative and cognitive institutionalization. The structures of mental health providers' minds and the values they hold dear cannot be legislated. The best that lawmakers can do is to populate the organizations with like-minded individuals, which Medicaid regulations do to a degree through their credentialization, especially at the higher reaches of organizations. That, along with reports and "vision statements," can work toward establishing values and cognitive scripts—but cannot force their internalization by managers or workers. Legislators are much more able to force regulative institutionalization. Regulating behavior and tying clear sanctions to noncompliance is a much more achievable goal. Over time, if compliance is achieved, perhaps patterned behavior could lead to the structuring of newer workers' minds (Berger and Luckmann 1966; Zucker 1977).

Of course, there may be reasons for policymakers avoiding regulative institutionalization. Intentional ambiguity can be useful, allowing deal-making, coalition building, and defusing of opposition (Baier, March, and Saetren 1986). Eschewing the nuts and bolts and instead endorsing platitudes and value statements allows policymakers to give the appearance of agreement without being held to account for the consequences of what implementing those statements might mean. To be fair, activists also find use in such ambiguity. Who can oppose harm reduction if there is no clear definition (Reinarman 2004)?

What the implementation of logics often comes down to is worker discretion. I described maximizing discretion as a key component of the clinical-professional logic, but in practice, the amount of discretion workers had in a given situation at Urban and Suburban was a result of how the competing logics involved were institutionalized. A relative lack of detailed regulative institutionalization allowed workers discretion in implementing the empowerment logic. At the same time, another logic—bureaucratic accountability—was also involved in many decisions, and this logic constrained workers' actions much more than the empowerment logic. Workers often opted for meeting the demands of bureaucratic accountability because the way was clearer and the consequences of not doing so were more dire. When logics conflict, those that are translated into more rigid standards are more likely to be followed (cf. Bryson 2005; Sosin 2010). The logic of bureaucratic accountability is an example par excellence, but we also saw that the community logic has—at least recently—been given more rigid implementation as well, at least when compared to the empowerment logic.

In the wake of tragedies such as the Sandy Hook massacre, there may be reluctance to allow people with severe mental illness to have a great deal of self-determination in care—such as the right to refuse treatment (Torrey 2008). Models of care exist, however, that do much more to institutionalize the empowerment logic in mental health care in other, perhaps more acceptable, ways. Noncompliance with regulative institutionalization often results in withdrawal of funding for providers. I have shown that the empowerment logic does not often have such regulatory backing. The self-directed care model (Center for Mental Health Services 2005; Cook et al. 2008) is a prime example of how to give it such heft. In systems organized along these lines, such as demonstration programs implemented in Florida, government funds follow the client and are used for services the client wants, from whichever provider the client chooses. Around half of the program's budget is required to be allocated to "traditional" behavioral services, and there is financial and professional oversight (Cook et al. 2008), but there is a great deal more client control of their treatment here than in traditional services—and this difference is ensconced in regulation.

Limitations and Qualifications

This study cannot be considered to represent the community mental health services system in its entirety. Despite the fact that readers of the study have commented that they could see the dynamics described here happening in a mental health care organization anywhere in the country, my observations were made in a restricted geographical area. Although there is a great deal of variation between the two sites, they are located in the same metropolitan region. Future research could undertake larger-scale studies to explore if these findings are borne out on a national or international scale.

In the effort to examine the dueling constraints involved in institutional fragmentation, my argument has underemphasized the ways institutional logics are constitutive—not simply limiting—of action (Sewell 1992). As was seen in the examples of informal labeling and practical empowerment, institutional logics in mental health care actually informed the actions that workers themselves chose to perform, even though those actions often did not take place in the way policymakers or stakeholders planned or desired.

As should be clear to the reader at this point, though this study no doubt considers different aspects of clinical work, it is a work of sociology, not a clinical evaluation of the two organizations. There were aspects of the clinical care at both organizations that did not receive much coverage within these pages. This is because they were secondary components that did not have much bearing on the dynamics I explored. Institutional fragmentation and worker adaptation to it doubtlessly affect clinical outcomes, but those effects were not a central focus of this study.

Finally, I have not attempted in this study to perform an exposé on the misguided actions or motivations of mental health workers or government bureaucrats. I sincerely believe that the vast majority of actions and motivations described here were directed at providing what those involved saw as work and services that would in some way better the lives of clients or other citizens. Nevertheless, in the course of so doing, high ideals can meet with hard realities in organizational life, and services may not be carried out in the hoped-for or expected way. The result should not cast a pall over the effort. I end with a quote from an admired scholar who saw a similar risk of misinterpretation of his study conducted over a half century ago: "While I . . . believe . . . that the corruption of ideals is easier than their fulfillment, and is in that sense more 'natural,' it does not follow that we should fail to treasure what is precarious or cease to strive for what is nobly conceived" (Selznick 1984 [1949]: x).

Notes

Chapter 1 Introduction

1. The organization's numerous residential programs were scattered in buildings throughout the neighborhood, each with its own staff. Though I conducted limited interviews and analyses of documents produced by and about these programs, the majority of the study focused on the case management and day programs.

Chapter 2 Logic and Constraint

1. Not every instance of doing "clinical" work necessarily meant that a worker was acting on this logic, as I describe it here. For instance, a manager at Suburban saw clinical value in workers learning to do things (such as gardening or learning to take public transportation) alongside clients, somewhat undercutting the expertise component of the logic.
2. Because Medicaid is a state-federal partnership program, regulations vary from state to state. Thus the particular set of regulations governing mental health services funded through Medicaid varies. Nevertheless, Medicaid is a major source of mental health funding for people with chronic mental illness nationally (Day 2006; Mechanic 2007), and so one can expect that rules governing its funding of mental health care are a major regulatory force throughout the country.
3. http://www.carf.org/consumer.aspx?Content=Content/ConsumerServices/cs01en. html&ID=1, accessed 3/19/2009. CARF has since removed the "consumer" section of its website (including that quoted here) and has replaced it with a section for the "public."
4. The actual name of the plan varied. This particular variant is my own creation and is used to refer to the tools used by both sites.
5. Scheid (2003) sees the concern with quality as having distinct origins from concerns with costs in mental health care, and Mendel, Scott, and colleagues (Mendel and Scott 2010; Scott et al. 2000) charted that cost concerns and quality concerns are rooted in distinct logics in health care. My research uncovered dynamics in which the two were tightly interwoven as different components of a unified logic that was focused on accountability for services provided, providing maximum quality at minimum cost.

Chapter 3 Diagnosis, Labeling, and Social Control

1. Rule-out diagnoses are given when a clinician believes that there is not enough information to confirm a diagnosis, but that the diagnosis exists as an alternative pending further information.
2. The *DSM IV* offers a multi-axial approach for assessing patients. Axis I focuses on clinical disorders, the most commonly assigned diagnoses. Axis II is restricted to personality disorders and mental retardation. Axis III deals with medical conditions, while Axis IV deals with psychosocial issues such as housing, education, or occupational problems. Finally, Axis V focuses on the Global Assessment of Function. The *DSM V* eliminates the multi-axial system.

3. Disorders acceptable for target population were the following: Schizophrenia, Schizophrenoform Disorder, Schizoaffective Disorder, Delusional Disorder, Shared Psychotic Disorder, Brief Psychotic Disorder, Psychotic Disorder Not Otherwise Specified, Bipolar Disorders, Cyclothymic Disorder, Major Depression, Obsessive-Compulsive Disorder, Anorexia Nervosa, and Bulimia Nervosa.

4. In addition to these criteria, requirements to qualify for certain services (such as housing funded by the federal Department of Housing and Urban Development) also included demonstrating homelessness or a lack of financial resources.

5. At Urban, which had a high proportion of clients dually diagnosed with both mental illness and substance abuse disorders, staff could at times label clients severely mentally ill based solely upon severe, prolonged substance abuse. For instance, one worker, Ivan, described a client with severe alcohol abuse problems in "non-clinical" terms as "a stone alcoholic." He said the client would probably die if he stopped drinking, even under medical supervision (field notes). However, clients were much less likely to be informally labeled severely mentally ill based on these criteria than they were based on symptoms of other clinical disorders.

6. I use a narrow conception of social control here. I refer simply to staff's efforts to ensure client compliance with organizational rules and routines. Broader conceptions might include attention to the ways that the institution of medicine—especially psychiatry—is itself an agent of social control, even when engaging in "therapeutic" practices (see Zola, "Medicine as an Institution of Social Control"; Conrad and Schneider, *Deviance and Medicalization*), or that social control is pervasive in all aspects of life (see, for instance, Horwitz, *Logic of Social Control*). Although I acknowledge the importance of the dynamics these alternative conceptions address, I purposefully avoid the broader issues in order to clearly home in on the maintenance of intra-organizational order.

Chapter 4   Empowerment Practice, Practical Empowerment

1. I thank Mark Peyrot for suggesting this term.

2. Though recorded before their book was released, this strategy appears to be a nice example of the "nudging" described by Thaler and Sunstein (2008).

3. This strategy resembles the strategy of seeking assent (rather than consent) that Anspach (1993) describes staff in infant intensive care units using with infants' parents.

Chapter 5   The Realities of Community Integration

1. As pointed out in an earlier chapter, an exception to this was Suburban's charging money for lunch, which clients could avoid paying by working in either preparing lunch or cleaning up afterward.

2. Near the end of my fieldwork, both organizations began to try to use a more formal tool to determine the level of independence and service need of clients: the Level of Care Utilization System published by the American Association of Community Psychiatrists (2000). The tool gauges numerous different domains of the clients' life: risk of harm, functional status, comorbidity with addiction and medical issues, environmental factors affecting mental health status, level of support, history of treatment, and current level of client engagement with treatment. Based on the formal numerical ratings on these criteria, the appropriate level of services are ranked on a six-level range from basic services (minimal involvement in services) to medically managed residential services (basically, hospitalization). The tool was just beginning to be considered and had not yet been formally implemented when I

ended my research, so it is unclear how it affected the implementation of the community logic. However, given the dynamics described in chapter 3 regarding official versus informal labels, and the way informal labels affected expectations here, there appears to be at least the potential that a similar bifurcation could occur in official versus informal labels regarding community integration.

Chapter 6 The Right Person for the Job

1. Another reason this issue was less explicitly addressed in my data was that during my time at Suburban, I was not as focused on this topic in my data gathering as I would come to be when I was collecting data at Urban.
2. I thank Matt Ezzell for this turn of phrase.
3. Alisa Lincoln, personal communication.

Chapter 7 Conclusion

1. In Scott's (2008) formulation, institutional logics belong in the cognitive type of institutionalization. However, both Scott himself (Scott et al. 2000) and others applying the perspective (Caronna 2004) have related logics to all three "pillars." I do so as well.

References

Abbott, Andrew Delano. 1988. *The System of Professions: An Essay on the Division of Expert Labor.* Chicago: University of Chicago Press.

Angell, Beth, Colleen A. Mahoney, and Noriko Ishibashi Martinez. 2006. "Promoting Treatment Adherence in Assertive Community Treatment." *Social Service Review* 80:485–526.

Anspach, Renee. 1993. *Deciding Who Lives: Fateful Choices in the Intensive-Care Nursery.* Berkeley: University of California Press.

Anthony, William A., E. Sally Rogers, and Marianne Farkas. 2003. "Research on Evidence-Based Practices: Future Directions in an Era of Recovery." *Community Mental Health Journal* 39, no. 2:101–114.

Appelbaum, Paul S., and Allison Redlich. 2006. "Use of Leverage Over Patients' Money to Promote Adherence to Psychiatric Treatment." *Journal of Nervous and Mental Disease* 194, no. 4:294–302.

Baier, V. E., J. E. March, and Harald Saetren. 1986. "Implementation and Ambiguity." *Scandinavian Journal of Management Studies* 2:197–212.

Baker, F., and H. C. Schulberg. 1967. "Development of a Community Mental Health Ideology Scale." *Community Mental Health Journal* 3:216–225.

Barley, Stephen R. "Coalface Institutionalism." 2008. In *The Sage Handbook of Organizational Institutionalism*, edited by R. Greenwood, C. Oliver, R. Suddaby, and K. Sahlin, 491–518. Thousand Oaks, CA: Sage.

Belknap, Ivan. 1956. *Human Problems of a State Mental Hospital.* New York: McGraw-Hill.

Bellack, Alan S. 2006. "Consumer and Scientific Models of Recovery in Schizophrenia: Concordance, Contrasts, and Implications." *Schizophrenia Bulletin* 32, no. 3:432–442.

Berger, Peter L., and Thomas Luckmann. 1966. *The Social Construction of Reality: A Treatise in the Sociology of Knowledge.* Garden City, NY: Anchor Books.

Binder, Amy. 2007. "For Love and Money: Organizations' Creative Responses to Multiple Environmental Logics." *Theory and Society* 36:547–571.

Bittner, E., and H. Garfinkle. 1967. "'Good' Organizational Reasons for 'Bad' Clinic Records." In *Studies in Ethnomethodology*, edited by H. Garfinkle, 186–207. Englewood Cliffs, NJ: Prentice Hall.

Bond, Gary R. 2004. "How Evidence-Based Practices Contribute to Community Integration." *Community Mental Health Journal* 40, no. 6:569–588.

Bourdieu, Pierre. 1977. *Outline of a Theory of Practice.* Cambridge: Cambridge University Press.

Braithwaite, John. 1989. *Crime, Shame, and Reintegration.* New York: Cambridge University Press.

Brown, J. D. 1991. "The Professional Ex: An Alternative for Exiting the Deviant Career." *Sociological Quarterly* 43, no. 2:219–230.

Brown, Phil. 1981. "The Mental Patients' Rights Movement and Mental Health Institutional Change." *International Journal of Health Services* 11, no. 4:523–540.

———. 1987. "Diagnostic Conflict and Contradiction in Psychiatry." *Journal of Health and Social Behavior* 28, no. 1:37–50.

Brown-Saracino, Japonica. 2010. *The Gentrification Debates.* New York: Routledge.

Bryson, Bethany Paige. 2005. *Making Multiculturalism: Boundaries and Meaning in U.S. English Departments.* Stanford, CA: Stanford University Press.

Caronna, Carol A. 2004. "The Misalignment of Institutional 'Pillars': Consequences for the U.S. Health Care Field." *Journal of Health and Social Behavior* 45 (Extra Issue):45–58.

Carter, P. L. 2006. "Straddling Boundaries: Identity, Culture, and School." *Sociology of Education* 79, no. 3:304–328.

Casalino, L. P. 2004. "Unfamiliar Tasks, Contested Jurisdictions: The Changing Organization Field of Medical Practice." *Journal of Health and Social Behavior* 45 (Extra Issue):59–75.

Clay, Sally, Bonnie Schell, Patrick W. Corrigan, and Ruth O. Ralph, eds. 2005. *On Our Own, Together: Peer Programs for People with Mental Illness.* 1st ed. Nashville: Vanderbilt University Press.

Cohen, Lizabeth. 2003. *A Consumers' Republic: The Politics of Mass Consumption in Postwar America.* 1st ed. New York: Knopf.

Comstock, D. L., T. R. Hammer, J. Strentzsch, K. Cannon, J. Parsons, and G. Salazar. 2008. "Relational-Cultural Theory: A Framework for Bridging Relational, Multicultural, and Social Justice Competencies." *Journal of Counseling & Development* 86:279–287.

Conrad, Peter, and Joseph W. Schneider. 1992. *Deviance and Medicalization: From Badness to Sickness.* Philadelphia: Temple University Press.

Cook, J. A., C. Russell, D. D. Grey, and J. A. Jonikas. 2008. "Economic Grand Rounds: A Self-Directed Care Model for Mental Health Recovery." *Psychiatric Rehabilitation Journal* 59:600–602.

Cook, J. A., and E. R. Wright. 1995. "Medical Sociology and the Study of Severe Mental Illness: Accomplishments and Directions for Future Research." *Journal of Health and Social Behavior* 35 (Extra Issue):95–114.

Costello, Carrie Yang. 2005. *Professional Identity Crisis: Race, Class, Gender, and Success at Professional Schools.* 1st ed. Nashville, TN: Vanderbilt University Press.

Cuddeback, G. S., and Joseph P. Morrissey. 2010. "Integrating Service Delivery Systems for Persons with a Severe Mental Illness." In *A Handbook for the Study of Mental Health: Social Contexts, Theories, and Systems,* edited by Teresa L. Scheid and Tony N. Brown, 510–528. New York: Cambridge University Press.

Davidson, Larry, and David Roe. 2007. "Recovery From versus Recovery In Serious Mental Illness: One Strategy for Lessening Confusion Plaguing Recovery." *Journal of Mental Health* 16, no. 4:459–470.

Day, S. L. 2006. "Issues in Medicaid Policy and System Transformation: Recommendations from the President's Commission." *Psychiatric Services* 57:1713–1718.

Dill, Ann E. P. 2001. *Managing to Care: Case Management and Service System Reform.* New York: Aldine de Gruyter.

DiMaggio, Paul J., and Walter W. Powell. 1983. "The Iron Cage Revisited: Institutional Isomorphism and Collective Rationality in Organizational Fields." *American Sociological Review* 48:147–160.

Dobransky, Kerry. 2009. "Help Me Help You: The Logic and Practice of Empowerment in Community Mental Health Services." PhD diss., Northwestern University.

Drake, Robert E., Susan M. Essock, Andrew Shaner, Kate B. Carey, Kenneth Minkoff, Lenore Kola, David Lynde, Fred C. Osher, Robin E. Clark, and Lawrence Rickards. 2001a. "Evidence-Based Practices—Implementing Dual Diagnosis Services for Clients with Severe Mental Illness." *Psychiatric Services: A Journal of the American Psychiatric Association* 52, no. 4:8.

Drake, Robert E., Howard H. Goldman, H. Stephen Leff, Anthony F. Lehman, Lisa Dixon, Kim T. Mueser, and William C. Torrey. 2001b. "Evidence-Based Practices—Implementing Evidence-Based Practices in Routine Mental Health Service Settings." *Psychiatric Services: A Journal of the American Psychiatric Association* 52, no. 2:4.

Du Bois, W.E.B. 1904. *The Souls of Black Folk.* Chicago: A. C. McClurg and Co.

Duneier, Mitchell, and Ovie Carter. 1999. *Sidewalk.* 1st ed. New York: Farrar, Straus and Giroux.

Emerson, Robert M., and Melvin Pollner. 1978. "Policies and Practices of Psychiatric Case Selection." *Sociology of Work and Occupations* 5:75–96.

Espeland, W. N., and B. I. Vannebo. 2007. "Accountability, Quantification, and Law." *Annual Review of Law and Social Science* 3:21–43.

Estroff, Sue E. 1981. *Making It Crazy: An Ethnography of Psychiatric Clients in an American Community.* Berkeley: University of California Press.

Floersch, Jerry. 2000. *Meds, Money, and Manners: The Case Management of Severe Mental Illness.* New York: Columbia University Press.

Free to Choose: Transforming Behavioral Health Care to Self-Direction. 2005. DHHS Publication No. SMA-05-3982. Rockville, MD: Center for Mental Health Services, Substance Abuse and Mental Health Services Administration.

Freidson, Eliot. 2001. *Professionalism: The Third Logic.* Cambridge: Polity.

Friedland, Roger, and Robert R. Alford. 1991. "Bringing Society Back In: Symbols, Practices, and Institutional Contradictions." In *The New Institutionalism in Organizational Analysis,* edited by Walter W. Powell and Paul J. DiMaggio, 232–263. Chicago: University of Chicago Press.

Gengler, Amanda M. 2012. "Defying (Dis)Empowerment in a Battered Women's Shelter: Moral Rhetorics, Intersectionality, and Processes of Control and Resistance." *Social Problems* 59, no. 4:501–521.

Goffman, Erving. 1961. *Asylums.* New York: Anchor Books.

Goldman, Howard H., and Joseph P. Morrissey. 1985. "The Alchemy of Mental Health Policy: Homelessness and the Fourth Cycle of Reform." *American Journal of Public Health* 75, no. 7:727–731.

Greenwood, R., Amalia Diaz, Stan Li, and Jose Lorente. 2010. "The Multiplicity of Institutional Logics and the Heterogeneity of Organizational Responses." *Organization Science* 21, no. 2:521–539.

Grob, Gerald N. 1991. *From Asylum to Community: Mental Health Policy in Modern America.* Princeton: Princeton University Press.

———. 1994. *The Mad among Us: A History of the Care of America's Mentally Ill.* New York: The Free Press.

Grob, Gerald N., and Howard H. Goldman. 2007. *The Dilemma of Federal Mental Health Policy: Radical Reform Or Incremental Change.* New Brunswick, NJ: Rutgers University Press.

Gulcur, Leyla. 2007. "Community Integration of Adults with Psychiatric Disabilities and Homelessness." *Community Mental Health Journal* 43, no. 3:211–228.

Hall, Wayne. 2007. "What's in a Name?" *Addiction* 102: 692.

Hallett, Tim. 2010. "The Myth Incarnate: Recoupling Processes, Turmoil, and Inhabited Institutions in an Urban Elementary School." *American Sociological Review* 75, no. 1:52–74.

Hallett, Tim, and Marc J. Ventresca. 2006. "Inhabited Institutions: Social Interactions and Organizational Forms in Gouldner's *Patterns of Industrial Bureaucracy*." *Theory and Society* 35:213–236.

Handler, Joel F. 1996. *Down from Bureaucracy: The Ambiguity of Privatization and Empowerment.* Princeton: Princeton University Press.

Hasenfeld, Yeheskel. 1986. "Community Mental Health Centers as Human Services Organizations." In *The Organization of Mental Health Services: Societal and Community Systems*, edited by W. Richard Scott and Bruce L. Black, 133–146. Beverly Hills, CA: Sage.

———. 2010a. "The Attributes of Human Services Organizations." In *Human Services as Complex Organizations*, edited by Yeheskel Hasenfeld, 9–32. Thousand Oaks, CA: Sage.

———. 2010b. "Theoretical Approaches to Human Service Organizations." In *Human Services as Complex Organizations*, edited by Yeheskel Hasenfeld, 33–57. Los Angeles: Sage.

Heimer, Carol A. 1999. "Competing Institutions: Law, Medicine, and Family in Neonatal Intensive Care." *Law and Society Review* 33, no. 1:17–66.

Heimer, Carol A., and Lisa R. Staffen. 1995. "Interdependence and Reintegrative Social Control: Labeling and Reforming 'Inappropriate' Parents in Neonatal Intensive Care Units." *American Sociological Review* 60:635–654.

———. 1998. *For the Sake of the Children: The Social Organization of Responsibility in the Hospital and the Home.* Chicago: University of Chicago Press.

Horwitz, Allan V. 1990. *The Logic of Social Control.* New York: Plenum Press.

Houghton Mifflin Company. 2000. *The American Heritage Children's Dictionary.* Boston: Houghton Mifflin Harcourt.

Institute of Medicine (U.S.). Committee on Quality of Health Care in America. 2001. *Crossing the Quality Chasm: A New Health System for the 21st Century.* Washington, DC: National Academy Press.

———. Committee on Crossing the Quality Chasm: Adaptation to Mental Health and Addictive Disorders. 2006. *Improving the Quality of Health Care for Mental and Substance-use Conditions.* Washington, DC: National Academies Press.

Jacobson, Nora. 2004. *In Recovery: The Making of Mental Health Policy.* 1st ed. Nashville, TN: Vanderbilt University Press.

Jutel, Annemarie. 2009. "Sociology of Diagnosis: A Preliminary Review." *Sociology of Health and Illness* 31, no. 2:278–299.

Jutel, Annemarie, and Sarah Nettleton. 2011. "Introduction: Towards a Sociology of Diagnosis: Reflections and Opportunities." *Social Science and Medicine* 73:793–800.

Kagan, Sharon Lynn, Peter R. Neville, and National Center for Service Integration. 1993. *Integrating Services for Children and Families: Understanding the Past to Shape the Future.* New Haven: Yale University Press.

Kahn, Alfred J., and Sheila B. Kamerman. 1992. *Integrating Services Integration: An Overview of Initiatives, Issues, and Possibilities.* New York: Cross-National Studies Research Program, Columbia University School of Social Work for the National Center for Children in Poverty, Columbia University School of Public Health.

Karp, David. 1986. "'You Can Take the Boy Out of Dorchester, but You Can't Take Dorchester Out of the Boy': Toward a Social Psychology of Mobility." *Symbolic Interaction* 9, no. 1:19–36.

Kirk, Stuart A., and Herb Kutchins. 1988. "Deliberate Misdiagnosis in Mental Health Practice." *Social Service Review* 62:225–237.

———. 1992. *The Selling of DSM: The Rhetoric of Science in Psychiatry.* New York: A. de Gruyter.

Lehman, Anthony F., L. T. Postrado, D. Roth, S. W. McNary, and Howard H. Goldman.

1994. "An Evaluation of Continuity of Care, Case Management, and Client Outcomes in the Robert Wood Johnson Program on Chronic Mental Illness." *Milbank Quarterly* 72, no. 1:105–122.

Linhorst, Donald M. 2006. *Empowering People with Severe Mental Illness: A Practical Guide.* New York: Oxford University Press.

Linhorst, Donald M., and Anne Eckert. 2003. "Conditions for Empowering People with Severe Mental Illness." *Social Service Review* 77, no. 2:279–305.

Lipsky, Michael. 1980. *Street-Level Bureaucracy: The Dilemmas of the Individual in Public Services.* New York: Russell Sage Foundation.

Lutterman, T., A. Berhane, B. Phelan, R. Shaw, and V. Rana. 2009. *Funding and Characteristics of State Mental Health Agencies, 2007.* Rockville, MD: Center for Mental Health Services, Substance Abuse and Mental Health Services Administration, US Department of Health and Human Services.

Manderscheid, R. W., M. J. Henderson, and D. Y. Brown. 2001. "Status of National Accountability Efforts at the Millennium." In *Mental Health, United States, 2000,* edited by R. W. Manderscheid and M. J. Henderson, 43–52. Washington, DC: Center for Mental Health Services, Substance Abuse and Mental Health Services Administration, US Department of Health and Human Services.

Mandiberg, J. M. 1999. "The Sword of Reform has Two Sharp Edges: Normalcy, Normalization, and the Destruction of the Social Group." *New Directions for Mental Health Services* 83:31–44.

March, James G., and Johan P. Olsen. 1976. *Ambiguity and Choice in Organizations.* Bergen, Norway: Universitetsforlaget.

Maynard-Moody, Steven, and Michael C. Musheno. 2003. *Cops, Teachers, Counselors: Stories from the Front Lines of Public Service.* Ann Arbor: University of Michigan Press.

McLean, Athena. 2000. "From Ex-Patient Alternatives to Consumer Options: Consequences of Consumerism for Psychiatric Consumers and the Ex-Patient Movement." *International Journal of Health Services* 30, no. 4:821–847.

———. 2010. "The Mental Health Consumers/Survivors Movement in the United States." In *Handbook for the Study of Mental Health: Social Contexts, Theories, and Systems,* edited by Teresa L. Scheid and Tony N. Brown, 461–477. New York: Cambridge University Press.

Mechanic, David. 2004. "The Rise and Fall of Managed Care." *Journal of Health and Social Behavior* 45 (Extra Issue):76–86.

———. 2007. *Mental Health and Social Policy: Beyond Managed Care.* 5th ed. Upper Saddle River, NJ: Allyn and Bacon.

Mendel, Peter, and W. Richard Scott. 2010. "Institutional Change and the Organization of Health Care." In *Handbook of Medical Sociology,* edited by C. Bird, P. Conrad, A. Fremont, and S. Timmermans, 249–269. Nashville, TN: Vanderbilt University Press.

Merton, Robert King. 1968. "The Matthew Effect in Science." *Science* 159:56–63.

Meyer, John W. 1986. "Institutional and Organizational Rationalization in the Mental Health System." In *The Organization of Mental Health Services: Societal and Community Systems,* edited by W. Richard Scott and Bruce L. Black, 215–227. Beverly Hills: Sage.

Meyer, John W., and Brian Rowan. 1977. "Institutionalized Organizations: Formal Structure as Myth and Ceremony." *American Journal of Sociology* 83, no. 2:340–363.

———. 1978. "The Structure of Educational Organizations." In *Environments and Organizations,* edited by Marshall W. Meyer, 78–109. San Francisco: Jossey-Bass.

Milazzo-Sayre, L. J., M. J. Henderson, R. W. Manderscheid, M. C. Bokossa, C. Evans, and A. A. Male. 2001. "Persons Treated in Specialty Mental Health Care Programs, United States, 1997." In *Mental Health, United States, 2000*, edited by R. W. Manderscheid and M. J. Henderson, 172–217. Washington, DC: Center for Mental Health Services, Substance Abuse and Mental Health Services Administration, US Department of Health and Human Services.

Miller, William R., and Stephen Rollnick, eds. 2002. *Motivational Interviewing: Preparing People for Change*. 2nd ed. New York: Guilford Press.

Monahan, John, Allison Redlich, Jeffrey Swanson, Pamela Clark Robbins, Paul S. Appelbaum, John Petrila, Henry J. Steadman, Marvin Swartz, Beth Angell, and Dale E. McNiel. 2005. "Use of Leverage to Improve Adherence to Psychiatric Treatment in the Community." *Psychiatric Services* 56, no. 1:37–44.

Morrissey, Joseph P., and Howard H. Goldman. 1986. "Care and Treatment of the Mentally Ill in the United States: Historical Developments and Reforms." *Annals of the American Academy of Political and Social Science* 484:12–27.

Obot, Isidore. 2007. "Harm Reduction: What Is It?" *Addiction* 102:691–692.

Ocasio, W. 1997. "Toward an Attention-Based View of the Firm." *Strategic Management Journal* 18:187–206.

Pager, Devah, and Lincoln Quillian. 2005. "Walking the Talk? What Employers Say versus What They Do." *American Sociological Review* 70, no. 3:355–380.

Parsons, Talcott. 1951. *The Social System*. Glencoe, IL: Free Press.

Peyrot, Mark. 1982. "Caseload Management: Choosing Suitable Clients in a Community Health Clinic Agency." *Social Problems* 30, no. 2:157–167.

———. 1985. "Coerced Voluntarism: The Micropolitics of Drug Treatment." *Urban Life* 13, no. 4:343–365.

———. 1991. "Institutional and Organizational Dynamics of Community-Based Drug Abuse Treatment." *Social Problems* 38, no. 1:20–33.

Peyser, H. 2001. "What Is Recovery? A Commentary." *Psychiatric Services* 52, no. 4:486–487.

Pfeffer, J., and Gerald R. Salancik. 2003 [1978]. *The External Control of Organizations: A Resource-Dependence Perspective*. Stanford, CA: Stanford University Press.

President's New Freedom Commission on Mental Health. 2003. *Achieving the Promise: Mental Health Care in America*. Washington, DC: United States Department of Health and Human Services, Substance Abuse and Mental Health Services Administration.

Ralph, Ruth O. 2005. "Verbal Definitions and Visual Models of Recovery: Focus on the Recovery Model." In *Recovery in Mental Illness: Broadening our Understanding of Wellness*, edited by Ruth O. Ralph and Patrick W. Corrigan, 131–146. Washington, DC: American Psychological Association.

Reinarman, Craig. 2004. "Public Health *and* Human Rights: The Virtues of Ambiguity." *International Journal of Drug Policy* 15:239–241.

Robbins, Pamela Clark, John Petrila, Stephanie LeMelle, and John Monahan. 2006. "The Use of Housing as Leverage to Increase Adherence to Psychiatric Treatment in the Community." *Administration and Policy in Mental Health and Mental Health Services Research* 33, no. 2:226–236.

Rosenhan, D. L. 1973. "On Being Sane in Insane Places." *Science* 179:250–258.

Rosenheck, R. A., Joseph P. Morrissey, J. Lam, M. Calloway, M. Johnsen, H. Goldman, F. Randolph, M. Blasinsky, A. Fontana, R. Calsin, and G. Teague. 1998. "Service System Integration, Access to Services, and Housing Outcomes in a Program for Homeless Persons with Severe Mental Illness." *American Journal of Public Health* 88, no. 11:1610–1615.

Rosenheck, R. A., J. Lam, J. P. Morrissey, M. O. Calloway, M. Stolar, F. Randolph, and ACCESS National Evaluation Team. 2002. "Service Systems Integration and Outcomes for Mentally Ill Homeless Persons in the ACCESS Program. Access to Community Care and Effective Services and Supports." *Psychiatric Services* 53, no. 8:958–966.

Roth, Julius A. 1972. "Some Contingencies of the Moral Evaluation of Clientele: The Case of the Hospital Emergency Service." *American Journal of Sociology* 77, no. 5:839–856.

Rothbard, A. B., S. Y. Min, E. Kuno, and Y. L. Wong. 2004. "Long-Term Effectiveness of the ACCESS Program in Linking Community Mental Health Services to Homeless Persons with Serious Mental Illness." *Journal of Behavioral Health Services & Research* 31, no. 4:441–449.

Scheid, Teresa L. 2003. "Managed Care and the Rationalization of Mental Health Services." *Journal of Health and Social Behavior* 44, no. 2:142–161.

———. 2004. *Tie a Knot and Hang On: Providing Mental Health Care in a Turbulent Environment.* New York: Aldine de Gruyter.

Scheid, Teresa L., and Greg Greenberg. 2007. "An Organizational Analysis of Mental Health Care." In *Mental Health, Social Mirror*, edited by William R. Avison, Jane D. McLeod, and B. A. Pescosolido, 379–406. New York: Springer.

Schlesinger, Mark, and Bradford Gray. 1999. "Institutional Change and Its Consequences for the Delivery of Mental Health Services." In *A Handbook for the Study of Mental Health: Social Contexts, Theories, and Systems*, edited by Allan V. Horwitz and Teresa L. Scheid, 427–448. Cambridge: Cambridge University Press.

Schneiberg, Marc, and Elisabeth Clemens. 2006. "The Typical Tools for the Job: Research Strategies in Institutional Analysis." *Sociological Theory* 24, no. 3:195–227.

Schutt, Russell K., and Stephen M. Goldfinger. 2011. *Homelessness, Housing, and Mental Illness.* Cambridge, MA: Harvard University Press.

Scott, Anne. 2012. "Authenticity Work: Mutuality and Boundaries in Peer Support." *Society and Mental Health* 1, no. 3:173–184.

Scott, W. Richard. 2008. *Institutions and Organizations: Ideas and Interests.* 3rd ed. Thousand Oaks, CA: Sage.

Scott, W. Richard, and John W. Meyer. 1991. "The Organization of Societal Sectors: Propositions and Early Evidence." In *The New Institutionalism in Organizational Analysis*, edited by Walter W. Powell and Paul J. DiMaggio, 108–140. Chicago: University of Chicago Press.

Scott, W. Richard, Martin Ruef, Carol A. Caronna, and Peter J. Mendel. 2000. *Institutional Change and Healthcare Organizations: From Professional Dominance to Managed Care.* Chicago: University of Chicago Press.

Segal, Steven P., and Uri Aviram. 1978. *The Mentally Ill in Community-Based Sheltered Care: A Study of Community Care and Social Integration.* New York: John Wiley and Sons.

Selznick, Philip. 1984 [1949]. *TVA and the Grass Roots: A Study of Politics and Organization.* Berkeley: University of California Press.

Sewell, W. H., Jr. 1992. "A Theory of Structure: Duality, Agency, Transformation." *American Journal of Sociology* 98:1–29.

Shorter, Edward. 1997. *A History of Psychiatry: From the Era of the Asylum to the Age of Prozac.* New York: John Wiley and Sons.

Smith, Brenda, and Stella Donovan. 2003. "Child Welfare Practice in Organizational and Institutional Context." *Social Service Review* 77, no. 4:541–563.

Sosin, Michael R. 2010. "Discretion in Human Service Organizations: Traditional and Institutional Perspectives." In *Human Services as Complex Organizations.* Edited by Yeheskel Hasenfeld, 381–403. Los Angeles: Sage.

Strathern, Marilyn. 2000. *Audit Cultures: Anthropological Studies in Accountability, Ethics, and the Academy.* London and New York: Routledge.

Strauss, Anselm L. 1987. *Qualitative Analysis for Social Scientists.* Cambridge: Cambridge University Press.

Strauss, Anselm L., Leonard Schatzman, Danuta Ehrlich, Rue Bucher, and Melvin Sabshin. 1963. "The Psychiatric Hospital and Its Negotiated Order." In *The Hospital in Modern Society.* Edited by Eliot Freidson, 147–169. New York: Free Press.

Tessler, Richard C., and Howard H. Goldman. 1982. *The Chronically Mentally Ill: Assessing Community Support Programs.* Cambridge, MA: Ballinger Publishing Company.

Thaler, Richard H., and Cass R. Sunstein. 2008. *Nudge: Improving Decisions about Health, Wealth, and Happiness.* New Haven: Yale University Press.

Thornton, Patricia H., and William Ocasio. 1999. "Institutional Logics and the Historical Contingency of Power: Executive Succession in the Higher Education Publishing Industry, 1958–1990." *American Journal of Sociology* 105, no. 3:801–843.

———. 2008. "Institutional Logics." In *The Sage Handbook of Organizational Institutionalism.* Edited by R. Greenwood, C. Oliver, R. Suddaby, and K. Sahlin, 99–129. Thousand Oaks, CA: Sage.

Thornton, Patricia H., William Ocasio, and Michael Lounsbury. 2012. *The Institutional Logics Perspective: A New Approach to Culture, Structure, and Process.* Oxford: Oxford University Press.

Timmermans, Stefan. 2010. "Evidence-Based Medicine: Sociological Explorations." In *Handbook of Medical Sociology.* Edited by C. Bird, P. Conrad, A. Fremont, and S. Timmermans, 309–323. Nashville, TN: Vanderbilt University Press.

Timmermans, Stefan, and Marc Berg. 2003. *The Gold Standard: The Challenge of Evidence-Based Medicine and Standardization in Health Care.* Philadelphia: Temple University Press.

Torrey, E. Fuller. 2008. *The Insanity Offense: How America's Failure to Treat the Seriously Mentally Ill Endangers Its Citizens.* New York: W. W. Norton.

Townsend, Elizabeth A. 1998. *Good Intentions Overruled: A Critique of Empowerment in the Routine Organization of Mental Health Services.* Toronto: University of Toronto Press.

Trends in Mental Health Systems Transformation: The States Respond.* 2006. DHHS Pub. No. (SMA) 05-4115. Rockville, MD: Center for Mental Health Services, Substance Abuse and Mental Health Services Administration.

Turner, Judith Clark, and William J. TenHoor. 1978. "The NIMH Community Support Program: Pilot Approach to a Needed Social Reform." *Schizophrenia Bulletin* 4, no. 3:319–348.

United States Congress House Committee on Government Reform Subcommittee on Criminal Justice Drug Policy and Human Resources. 2005. *Harm Reduction or Harm Maintenance: Is There Such a Thing as Safe Drug Abuse?* Hearing before the Subcommittee on Criminal Justice, Drug Policy, and Human Resources of the Committee on Government Reform, House of Representatives, One Hundred Ninth Congress, First Session, February 16. Washington, DC: GPO.

Venkatesh, Sudhir Alladi. 2006. *Off the Books: The Underground Economy of the Urban Poor.* Cambridge, MA: Harvard University Press.

Watkins-Hayes, Celeste. 2009. *The New Welfare Bureaucrats: Entanglements of Race, Class, and Policy Reform.* Chicago: University of Chicago Press.

Wilson, Mitchell. 1993. "DSM-III and the Transformation of American Psychiatry: A History." *American Journal of Psychiatry* 150, no. 3:399–410.

Zdanowicz, Mary T. 2006. "Recovery and Coercion: Reconciling Two Hotbutton Terms." *Catalyst* Spring:1–16.

Zola, I. K. 1972. "Medicine as an Institution of Social Control." *Sociological Review* 20.

Zucker, Lynne G. 1977. "The Role of Institutionalization in Cultural Persistence." *American Sociological Review* 42, no. 5:726–743.

Index

ACCESS program (Access to Community Care and Effective Services), 6
ACT. *See* assertive community treatment
advocacy, 29–30
allocating choice, 93–95
American Association of Community Psychiatrists, 154n2 (chap. 5)
Annie E. Casey Foundation, xi
assertive community treatment (ACT), 25, 36, 40, 47, 112, 124
auditing, 2, 43, 46, 90, 92; by CARF, 32, 50; by the state, 34, 41, 124
Aviram, Uri, 107

Baker, Frank, 36
Belknap, Ivan, 57
billing, 8, 25, 40, 46, 47, 97, 146; push to maximize, 3, 7, 49, 60–62, 91–92, 95–97. *See also* workers, mental health: productivity of
Binder, Amy, 147–148
boundaries, professional, 122, 130–137
Bourdieu, Pierre, 105
Brown, J. D., 126
bureaucratic accountability, logic of, xii, 7–8, 10, 43–45, 145, 147, 148; and empowerment practice, 89–99; institutionalization of, 11, 49–51, 89–90, 146, 150; and labeling clients, 60–63, 75; main components of, 45–49

CARF. *See* Commission on the Accreditation of Rehabilitation Facilities
choosing dependence, 113–120, 145. *See also* clients, mental health: independence of
clients, mental health: advisory councils for, 34–35, 81–82; as consumers, 7, 10, 26, 31, 125; families of, 38, 105, 109, 120; functioning of, 61, 64, 68; independence of, 3, 38–43, 87, 105–106, 113–120; reasons for seeking services, 58–59, 94; resources of, 82–89, 93, 95, 97–99, 107–110; self-determination of, 27–29, 30–33, 78–99, 114–119, 146, 150; stigmatization of, 27, 57–58, 62, 108, 111, 120; terminology used to address, xiii; treatment history of, 57–58
clinical-professional logic, xii, 7–8, 20–21, 145, 148, 150; in diagnosing clients, 55, 57, 61, 75, 147; institutionalization of, 24–26, 124–125; main components of, 21–24; in staffing, 123–144
Commission on the Accreditation of Rehabilitation Facilities (CARF), 31–32, 34–36, 47, 49–51, 81–82, 153n3

community logic, xii, 3, 7–8, 102–107, 145–146, 148; history of, 36–37; institutionalization of, 40–43, 115, 150; main components of, 37–40. *See also* integration, social/community
Community Mental Health Center Act/Program, 4
community mental health ideology, 36
community support: as federal program, 5, 36–37, 112; as state Medicaid mental health service, 36, 40–41, 47, 115, 124
cost containment, 8, 10, 43–44, 47, 51, 145
Costello, Carrie Yang, 136

decoupling, 147
deinstitutionalization, 5, 36
demographics, of workers and clients, 12, 14, 125–130, 135–137, 138–139, 142–144
diagnosis, psychiatric, 53–55, 67; informal, 64–75, 117–120, 154n5; and medical necessity, 60, 75; official, 55–65, 69, 74–75
Diagnostic and Statistical Manual of Mental Disorders (*DSM*), 25, 55, 60–61, 74, 153n2 (chap. 3)
dialectical behavior therapy, 47–48
documentation, 43, 45–46, 49, 50, 60, 88, 90–91
dual diagnosis (substance abuse and mental illness), services for, 6, 31, 62
Du Bois, W.E.B., 136

empowerment logic, xii, 7–8, 10, 26–27, 145, 148; ambiguity surrounding, 27, 78–83, 86, 115; and empowerment practice, 77–99, 114–120, 133–137; institutionalization of, 11, 30–36, 90, 115, 124–125, 146, 150; main components of, 27–30; and practical empowerment, 93–99, 151; in staffing, 123–129, 139–144. *See also* harm reduction; recovery, mental health
evidence-based practice, 2, 6, 47–48, 50–51. *See also* assertive community treatment; dialectical behavior therapy; illness management and recovery; vocational services: supported employment as

gender. *See* demographics, of workers and clients
Goffman, Erving, 56, 86
Goldfinger, Stephen, 29, 36, 113
government: federal, 4–5, 34; state (*see* state government)

habitus, of clients, 105–106, 114
harm reduction, 31, 33, 114; ambiguity surrounding, 27, 80–81, 88, 150

state government, 4, 10–11; mental health financing by, 2, 10, 34, 40–41, 47–48, 50, 60–62, 64; mental health regulation instituted by, 30, 34, 40–41, 47, 89, 113, 137, 140, 142–143. *See also* Medicaid
steering choice, 96–98
Strauss, Anselm, 9, 12, 133, 142
substance abuse. *See* dual diagnosis
Substance Abuse and Mental Health Services Administration, U.S. *See* SAMHSA
Suburban (field site), 41–42, 65, 84–86, 109, 143; description, 14–15; parent organization Wellness, 3, 10, 30, 77, 79–81, 84, 85, 101, 112, 125
symptoms, of mental illness, 29, 53–55, 60, 114, 119; client disruptions viewed as, 64–74, 93; feigned/exaggerated, 59, 69, 118

Townsend, Elizabeth, 37, 92
treatment plans, personalized, 34–36, 45, 81, 82, 87–88, 103, 114

Urban (field site), 41–42, 65, 86–89, 108, 143–144; description, 12–14
U.S. Department of Housing and Urban Development. *See* HUD

vocational services, 10, 31, 81; as social (vs. health) services, 5, 59–60; at Suburban, 7, 14–15, 38–39, 63, 85, supported employment as, 48, 101

Watkins-Hayes, Celeste, 21, 60, 89–90, 98, 129–130, 135
work crews, client, 79–80
workers, mental health: classifications of, 24–25, 124, 135, 140; discretion of, 21–22, 65, 82, 85–86, 150; education/training of, 20, 22, 24–26, 123–129, 143, 149; expertise of, 3, 23–26, 65, 123–129; jurisdiction of, 22–25; personas of, 130–137, 141; and productivity, 48–50, 60, 77–78, 91–93
workshop, sheltered, 14, 38, 101, 116, 137–138

About the Author

Kerry Dobransky received his PhD from Northwestern University. He is an assistant professor of sociology at James Madison University. His research focuses on health, illness, and disability; health care; organizations; and ICTs. Dr. Dobransky has published his work in journals such as *Social Science and Medicine*, *Advances in Medical Sociology*, and *Health Communication*. This is his first book.

Available titles in the Critical Issues in Health and Medicine series: